Multi-Trillion Dollar

U.S. Healthcare To 2020

Gold Rush

EDMUND L. VALENTINE

MMC International Publishing

Printed in the United States of America

10 09 08 07 06   5 4 3 2 1

Library of Congress Cataloging-in-Publication Data:

Valentine, Edmund L., 1946
Multi-Trillion Dollar U.S. Healthcare To 2020 Gold Rush ; Edmund L. Valentine
p. cm.
Includes Index
ISBN 09844047808 (paper)
ISBN-13 978-0-9840478-0-2 (paper)
1. Medical care – Technological innovations. 2. Medical care – Cost effectiveness.
3. Value analysis – Cost control. 4. U.S. healthcare. 5. Healthcare – competition.

ISBN: 0984047808
ISBN-13: 978-0-9840478-0-2
LCCN: 2011942966

DEDICATION

This book is dedicated to Kathie Valentine without whose support this book would never have been written.

CONTENTS

PREFACE

The 2012 through 2020 period presents companies and investors with unprecedented opportunities to create wealth. The Patient Protection and Affordable Care Act (PPACA), which contains provisions pioneered by both Republicans and Democrats, is the single largest technology stimulus, innovation implementation and development, job creation, and waste elimination legislation in the history of the United States (U.S.). PPACA is capitalizing on four major trends: 1) increasing demand, 2) new enabling technologies, 3) innovation, and 4) an imperative to contain increasing healthcare costs. If not contained, healthcare expenditures will decrease American's standard of living and ability to compete on a global basis. Implementation will result in market driven revolutionary change throughout every segment of the $2.6 trillion (17.3% of the U.S. 2010 gross domestic product, GDP) U.S. healthcare system (slightly larger than the GDP of the U.K.). It will cause a cultural shift within healthcare which will affect how each of the 17 million U.S. healthcare workers view and do their jobs. In the process, it will decrease inefficiencies/waste and create significant corporate and personal wealth.

Profit sharing through the elimination of over $1 trillion in annual U.S. healthcare system inefficiencies/waste is available ($12.1 trillion between 2012 and 2020). This is equal to about 10% annually of the U.S. GDP. To profit, industry participants are investing in new technologies, innovations and capabilities, creating new companies, increasing efficiencies, and eliminating waste. They are and will be creating jobs, products and services. Many of the products and services will serve customers worldwide, prompting job growth. History has shown that these periods of industry discontinuities result in: 1) lower consumer costs, 2) industry consolidations, 3) wealth creation for the leading companies in each major industry sector, and 4) create considerable wealth for investors/stockholders.

Industry participants change in anticipation of legislation and regulation. As a result, the direction for each of the respective industry segments started to be transformed prior to the March 23, 2010 passage of PPACA. The general direction has been set. The level of impact, the speed and degree of change, and success will in part be dependent upon implementing regulations. The changes will occur regardless of the political positioning between the Republican and Democratic legislators.

This book presents the major enabling technologies and innovations, the reason why passage of PPACA and related legislation and regulation was and will be needed. While not designed to recommend investments, the leading companies in each major U.S. healthcare industry segment are listed. The reader will also get insights relative to the respective industry strategic drivers and their implications for each of the major industry segments. Healthcare is replete with emerging, growth, maturing and mature industry segments. Each represents different levels of investment risk, potential growth, and stock price appreciation.

1 INTRODUCTION

U.S. healthcare represents a multi-trillion dollar wealth creation opportunity.

The 2012 through 2020 timeframe represents a period of unprecedented opportunity to create personal and corporate wealth. Passage of the American Recovery and Reinvestment Act of 2009 (ARRA) on February 17, 2009 and the Patient Protection and Affordable Care Act (PPACA) on March 23, 2010 has launched a period of intense healthcare innovation, change and industry discontinuity. History has shown that these are the times where investments in those companies that come to dominate their respective industries create significant returns/wealth for their stockholders.

Industry threats and opportunities foster change for gain or survival. The growing older population with longer life spans and an increasing number of chronic conditions will increasingly fuel demand for all types of health related products and services. Elimination of over $1 trillion in annual healthcare waste (about 10% of the 2010 United States Gross Domestic Product, GDP) through: 1) the implementation and/or creation of new technologies, 2) innovation in new ways of doing things to eliminate cost while increasing the quality of care, and 3) shifting unproductive expenditures into cost-effective products and services represents such an opportunity.

All U.S. healthcare industry participants, and their 17 million employees (about the population of Michigan), will be working to extract costs from the growing $2.6 Trillion (2010) healthcare system (slightly larger than the GDP of the United Kingdom) in order to share in the cost savings. The only certainties are that change will occur, a cultural shift of unprecedented size will have to take place, and some industry participants will prosper while others will be acquired, merged or driven out of business.

The U.S. healthcare system has gone through significant transformational change over the past 25 to 50 years, but more dramatic change lies ahead. What will occur and the direction of change can be seen in historic industry Lifecycles, e.g., horse-drawn wagons, buggy whips, cars, transistors, hardware stores, computers, picture film, etc. Healthcare is comprised of a myriad of industries, each in different stages of their respective industry Lifecycles. This book will present observations regarding each major sector.

PPACA is the biggest technology stimulus and job creation legislation in the history of the U.S.

PPACA is capitalizing on four major trends: 1) increasing demand, 2) new technologies, 3) innovation, and 4) an imperative to contain healthcare costs. Implementation is designed to be accomplished in 92 distinct but coordinated steps orchestrated to use grants, incentives, penalties, and market forces/competition to effectuate change. Implementation began in 2010 and is scheduled to be completed in 2018. To profit, industry participants are investing in new technologies and innovations, increasing efficiencies, and eliminating waste. They are and will be creating jobs, products and services. Many of the products and services will serve customers worldwide. PPACA is the single largest technology development, job creation, and waste elimination program in the history of the United States - and it is U.S. Federal Budget neutral. The level of impact, the speed and degree of change, and the level of success will be dependent upon implementing regulation. The changes will occur regardless of the political positioning between the Republican and Democratic legislators.

A number of U.S. healthcare transformational themes will be playing out over the next ten years.

There are a number of U.S. healthcare transformational themes playing out over the next ten years. The implications are profound and will not leave any segment of healthcare untouched. The impact will be industry segment and company specific.

Transformational Themes

From	To
Volume	Accountable Care
Duplicative Care	Coordinated Care
Emergency Care	Preventative Care
Procedures	Outcomes
Subjective	Objective
Drugs	Outcomes
Vertical Integration	Integration/Collaboration
Fragmented Care	Coordinated Care
Price	Value
Secretive	Collaborative
Data	Megadata
Insurance	Universal Coverage
Status Quo	Innovation
Evolutionary Change	Revolutionary Change
Reactive	Preventative
Passive	Involved
Ignorance	Educated
Guarded	Transparency
Independent	Interdependent
Computers and Servers	Cloud Computing
Independent Systems	Interactive Systems

Source: MMC International.

How To Read The Book

This book is designed for both a quick read and for a more detailed analysis. For a top line view, read the titles highlighted in bold and the black text following the top line. For a more detailed understanding, review the page graphics/content and the blue text. The source(s) of the information is listed on each page.

2 NEW ENABLING TECHNOLOGIES

Convergence of five technologies will enable the transformation of U.S. healthcare

Technology will enable innovations that will impact all healthcare segments/stakeholders. Where, when, how, and by whom patients are screened, diagnosed, treated, managed, and monitored will be transformed. How care is purchased and compensated will be fundamentally changed. How products are developed, marketed, evaluated, approved for reimbursement, purchased and utilized will be redefined over the next ten years. The number and type of intermediaries and their roles will be driven by measured cost effectiveness. All empowered by a myriad of new technologies and innovations enabled by the convergence of five technologies, computer hardware, software, the Internet, Wi-Fi, and genomics.

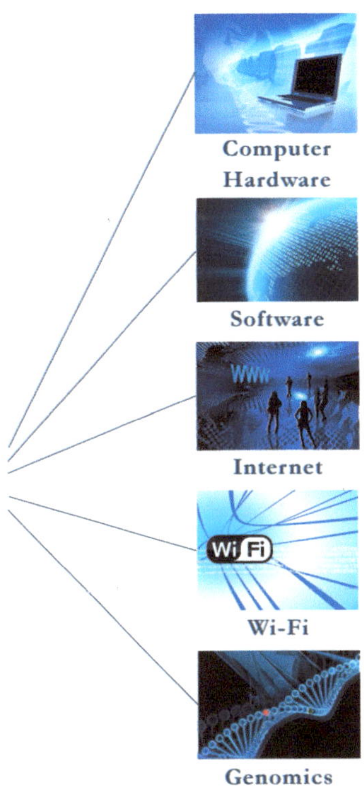

Source: MMC International.

- All the technologies benefit from economies of scale.
    - Costs decrease as volume/utilization increases.
    - Features and benefits increase, due to competition, while costs decrease.

- A myriad of things have to come together to move a technology from the laboratory to the market. Thereafter, other factors have to come into place to move the product from a few users to general adoption. These factors are indicators of how fast a market is likely to grow for a specific product or service.
    - Manufacturing has to be scaled up.
    - Industry standards have to be established.
    - Enabling legislation and policies have to be in place.
    - Reliability has to be proven.
    - Operation has to become more user friendly/simplified.
    - Price has to become cost effective.
    - Value to the user has to be established.
    - Reimbursement and/or value to the patient have to be provided.

Interoperable electronic health records (EHRs) will enable the revolutionary transformation of healthcare.

Deployment of Interoperable Electronic Health Records (EHRs) and a National Health Information Network (NHIN), together, will enable the revolutionary transformation of the U.S. healthcare system between 2010 and 2020. EHRs will decrease duplicative care, enable health outcomes research, and provide better continuity of care.

Electronic Patient Records (EMR, EHR, PHR)			
Electronic Medical Records (EMR)	**Electronic Health Records (HER)**	**Patient Health Record (PHR)**	
An electronic record of health-related information on an individual that can be created, gathered, managed and consulted by authorized clinicians and staff within one health care organization.	An electronic record of health-related information on an individual that conforms to nationally recognized interoperability standards and that can be created, managed, and consulted by authorized clinicians and staff across more than one health care organization.	An electronic record of health-related information on an individual that conforms to nationally recognized interoperability standards that can be drawn from multiple sources while being managed, shared, and controlled by the individual.	**Referred to As EHRs**

National Health Information Network (NHIN)			
Health Information Exchange (HIE)	**Health Information Organization (HIO)**	**Regional Health Information Organization (RHIO)**	
The electronic movement of health-related information among organizations according to nationally recognized standards.	An organization that oversees and governs the exchange of health-related information according to nationally recognized standards.	A health information organization that brings together health stakeholders within a defined geographic area and governs health information exchange among them for the purpose of improving health and care in the community.	**Referred to As the NHIN**

Sample Exchange and Patient Record Customers

Providers	
Physicians	629,000
Medical Laboratories	15,225
Radiology Groups	4,450
Hospitals	5,398
Nursing Homes	20,858
Home Healthcare Agencies	7,184
Pharmacies	61,101
Insurance Companies	1,300
Data Users	
Health Insurance Plans	1,300
Public Health/Medicare/Medicaid	>100
Disease Management Companies	~
Pharmaceutical Companies	~
Device Companies	~
Market Research Companies	~
Individuals	>307,000,000

Source: MMC International

Every hospital can have ≥200 different computer systems that have to be integrated. The majority of hospital implementations will have to be scrapped or totally reworked. Most physicians' offices, if they have an EHR system, will have to upgrade. All require billions in investments between now and 2020.

Everything is in place for the implementation of a national health information network (NHIN).

All the pieces are in place for the implementation of a National Health Information Network (NHIN): legislation, regulations, standards, incentives, financial support, software, networks, and examples of successful regional implementations.

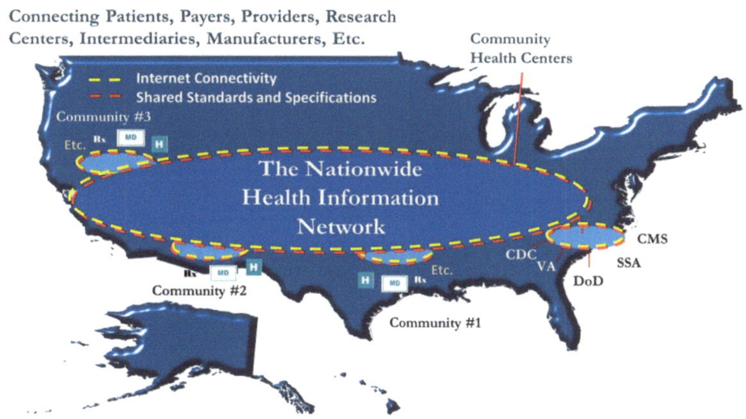

Legislation

- ARRA (American Recovery and Reinvestment Act of 2009)
  - Statutory Basis for the Medicare & Medicaid EHR (electronic health record) Incentive Programs.
  - The HITECH Act (Health Information Technology for Economic and Clinical Health Act), part of ARRA, amended several sections of the Social Security Act (SSA) and in doing so established the availability of incentive payments to eligible professionals and eligible hospitals to promote the adoption and "meaningful use" of interoperable health information technology (HIT).

Standards and Protocols

- The Nationwide Health Information Network, overseen by the Office of the National Coordinator for Health Information Technology, is a collection of standards, protocols, legal agreements, specifications and services designed to promote the development of a national infrastructure to support the secure exchange of health information over the Internet.

Financial Support

- Adoption of health information exchanges is expected to grow as a result of the passage of the 2009 ARRA and the 2010 PPACA. As of March 2010, 56 federal grants totaling $548 million had been awarded to states to facilitate and expand the secure electronic movement and use of health information among organizations, using nationally recognized standards.

ARRA incentives/penalties will drive the adoption of EHRs through 2015, operations through 2020.

In 2009, ARRA set aside $36 Billion to promote the "Meaningful Use" of "Qualified EHRs[1]" - $6.4 million in financial support for each hospital, and between $44,000.00 and $63,750.00 for each physician to implement EHRs. In order to receive reimbursements and avoid penalties in the form of reduced Medicare payments, EHRs must meet the meaningful use standards by 2015. Most hospitals and physicians contract IT vendors to assist in implementation.

- On July 13, 2010, the final e-health "meaningful use" rules were released[2].
  - Meaningful use is defined by a growing list of required features and capabilities that must be implemented in order to benefit from incentive payments as follows:

First Payment Year	Payment Year				
	2011	2012	2013	2014	2015
2011	Stage 1	Stage 1	Stage 2	Stage 2	TBD
2012		Stage 1	Stage 1	Stage 2	TBD
2013			Stage 1	Stage 1	TBD
2014				Stage 1	TBD

The final rule states: 'We expect that Stage 2 meaningful use requirements will include rigorous expectations for health information exchange...providers will electronically transmit patient care summaries to support transitions in care across unaffiliated providers, setting, and EHR systems.'

- Incentive payments will be made annually from 2011 through 2015.
  - Hospitals are eligible for up to $6.4 million to defray IT costs associated with deploying EMR technology.
  - Private practice clinicians can receive up to $44,000.00 per doctor in reimbursement funds through Medicare or $63,750.00 per doctor under Medicaid beginning in 2011.
  - Some insurance companies began offering similar incentives to get physicians to implement EHRs.

- In order to receive reimbursements and avoid penalties in the form of reduced Medicare payments, EHRs must meet the meaningful use standards by 2015.

1 EHR = Electronic Health Record; EMR = Electronic Medical Record; PHR = Patient Health Record. All are used interchangeably.
2 Released by the Department of Health and Human Services, Centers for Medicare & Medicaid Services, 42 CFR Parts 412, 413, 422, and 495, CMS-0033-F, RIN 0938-AP78, Medicare and Medicaid Programs; Electronic Health Record Incentive Program, Final rule.
TBD = to be determined.

EHR/NHIN industry software and support revenues are between $11.5 and $18.0 billion annually.

In 2010, there were 193 exchanges in development and 384 EHR vendors. The combined potential annual software sales and support fees for this emerging industry are between $11.5 and $18.0 Billion. The U.S. EHR market is 44% of the way to becoming consolidated.

National Health Information Network (NHIN)			Annual U.S. Revenues (In $ Billions)
Health Information Exchange (HIE)	Health Information Organization (HIO)	Regional Health Information Organization (RHIO)	$3.5 - $10.0 (Potential
Electronic Patient Records (EMR, EHR, PHR)			
Electronic Medical Records (EMR)	Electronic Health Records (HER)	Patient Health Record (PHR)	$3.5 - $10.0 (Potential

Market Leaders	Other Market Participants	
• Cerner	• CostFlex Systems	• CPSI
• GE	• Epic	• GE/IDX/Centricity
• Eclipsys	• Hyperion Solutions	• iSoft
• Siemens	• Kodak Health Group	• Lawson
	• Misys Healthcare Systems	• Meditech
	• mTuitive	• QuadraMed
	• SCC Soft Computer	• 365 Others

Source: MMC International.

Companies such as Allscripts (Eclipsys), Epic and Cerner could well be targets for larger companies like I.B.M., Microsoft, Oracle and McKesson that are looking to buy health information-technology specialists to grab market share.

NHIN and HER Industry Lifecycles

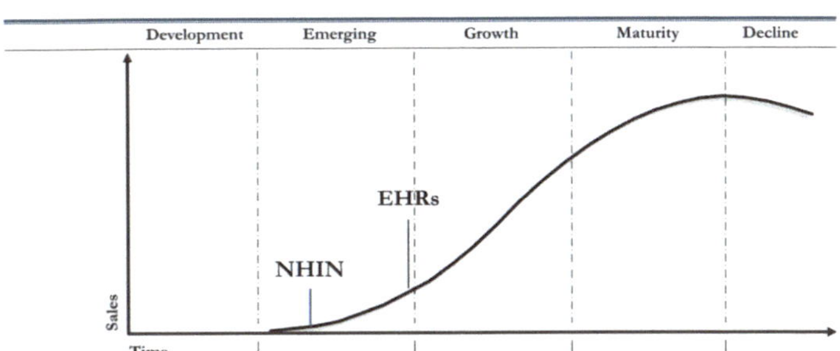

	Development	Emerging	Growth	Maturity	Decline
Risk	Medium	High / Medium	Medium / Low	Low / High	Low
Strategy	Develop Product Portfolio	Secure Market Position	Capture Dominant Market Position	Redeploy Resources (Higher Return Areas)	Focus on Free Cash Flows
Resource Allocation	Invest	Invest	Invest	Maintain/Harvest	Harvest

Source: MMC International

The U.S. EHR market is 44% of the way to becoming consolidated.

The personal genome promises to revolutionize how diseases are diagnosed, treated and managed.

The personal genome promises to revolutionize how diseases are defined, diagnosed, when and how they are treated and how they are managed. Personal genomic information will begin going mainstream over the next ten years.

The Shrinking Cost of DNA Sequencing
The $1,000 Genome

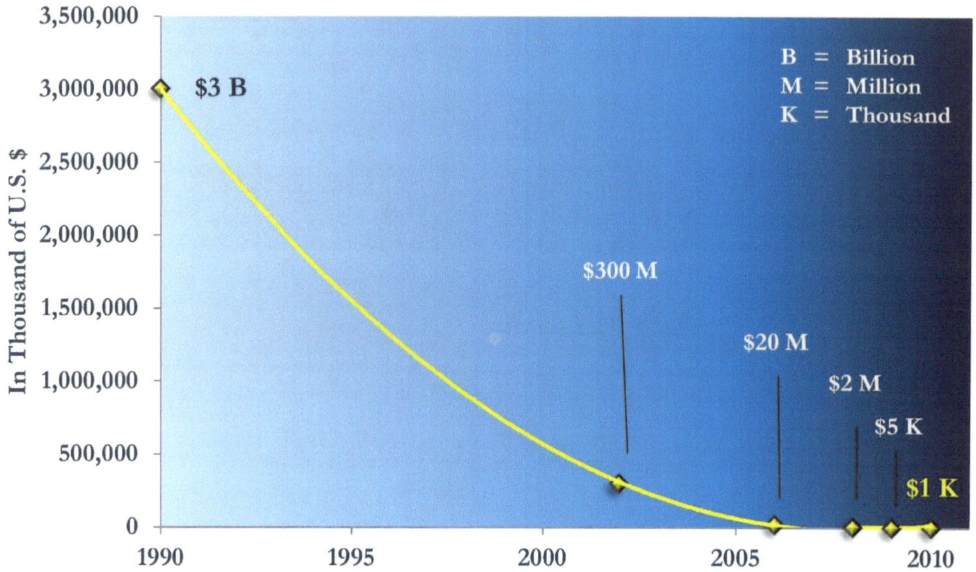

Sources: Wheeler DA et al., Nature 2008; 452:872-6; Mardis E. Genome Biology 2006; 7:112; Keim B. Wired Science October 06, 2008; The 2009 and 2010 values are projected. Cost of complete genome sequencing in April 2009 was $60,000 (Applied Biosystems); various Reports and MMC International.

The ability to profile the structure, sequence, and expression levels of genes, proteins, and metabolites is beginning to and will redefine how diseases are classified and treatments are selected. What was once thought to be a single disease characterized by a common set of physical signs and symptoms may be several distinct conditions, or it could be a single disease with a spectrum of treatment options, depending on the risk profile of the individual patient. For example, in the 1920s there were only two blood cancers, leukemia and lymphoma. Today, cellular and genetic analysis can distinguish 38 types of leukemia and 51 types of lymphoma. As a result, survival rates for many of the subtypes have improved from 0% to as high as 90%.

To be clinically useful, the patient's individual "Genome" needs to become part of his/her electronic medical record so that it can be compared with large-scale clinical outcomes information to predict risks and responses to treatments.

Large-scale population studies to link genetic and molecular signatures of disease and its treatments are required to make genetic sequencing a useful clinical tool. A number of government, academic and industry projects to generate publicly available data and frameworks to support large-scale genome-wide disease associations are under way (e.g., International HapMap Project; the Database of genotype and Phenotype (dbGAP); the Genetic Association Information Network (GAIN); The Biomarkers Consortium; the Genes, Environment and Health Initiative; The Cancer Genome Atlas; and the Serious Adverse Events Consortium).

Genomics will explode between 2012 and 2020.

Genomics, which is an emerging technology, is like the Internet in the early 1990's. It is an enabling technology with vast untapped potential and a myriad of applications, many which are unknown today. Genomics information will explode between 2012 and 2020. It will unleash an unprecedented amount of clinical information that will result in new products, change how drugs are developed, how diseases are classified, how and when diseases are treated, improve efficacy, reduce side effects, improve outcomes, and reduce healthcare costs. The true value of the human genome will begin to materialize when individuals' personal genome becomes part of their EHR. More detailed diagnoses and treatment information, in part enabled by the adoption of ICD-10 codes in 2013, will enable acceleration towards truly personalized medicine.

The Human Genome Project remains one of the largest single investigational projects in modern science.

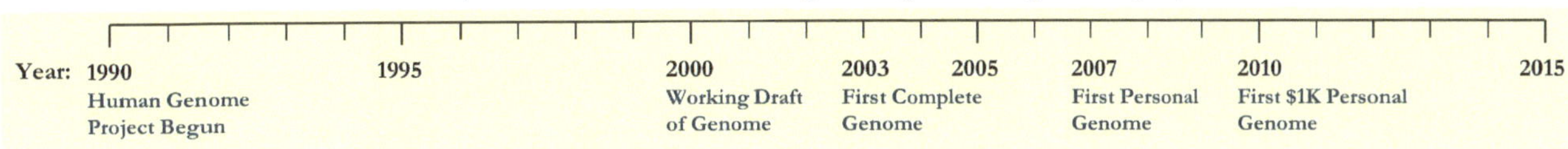

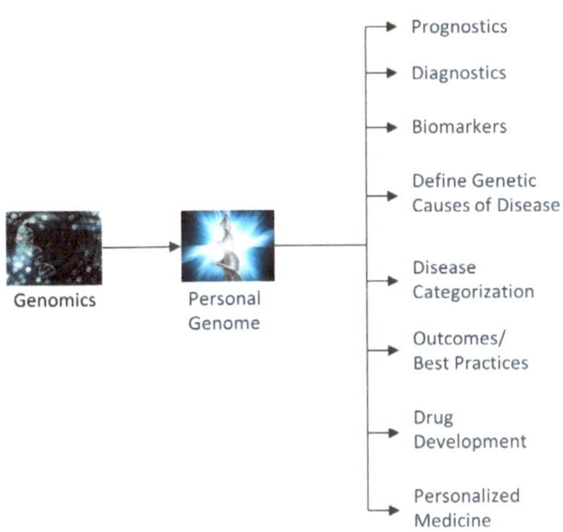

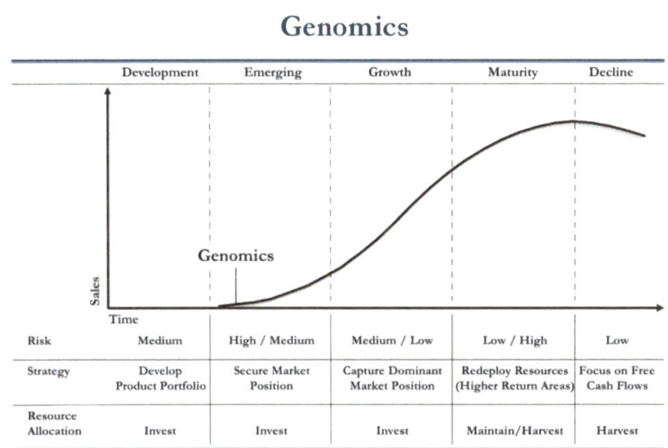

Source: MMC International

The following is an alphabetical list of companies competing to develop a full genome sequencing platform that is commercially robust for both research and clinical use.

- 454 Life Sciences
- BioNanomatrix
- Complete Genomics
- Genome Corporation
- Helicos Biosciences
- Illumina
- Intelligent Bio-Systems
- ION Torrent Systems
- Knome
- Pacific Biosciences
- Sequenom

The emerging $3 billion Pharmacogenomics testing market will grow at ≥45% annually.

Pharmacogenomics is an emerging $3 Billion, 2009, testing market, which has been growing at ≥45% annually. It will continue to enable the move toward personalized medicine and more cost-effective medication management. On average, marketed drugs only work in about half of the people who take them. Genomic biomarkers can play an important role in identifying responders and non-responders, avoiding toxicity and adjusting the dosage of drugs to optimize their efficacy and safety.

Pharmacogenomics

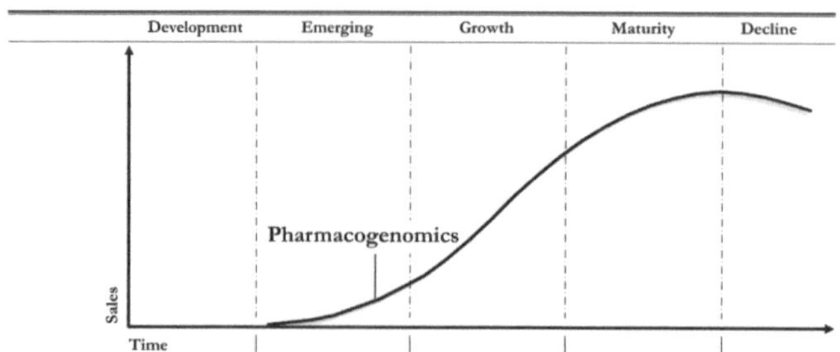

	Development	Emerging	Growth	Maturity	Decline
Risk	Medium	High / Medium	Medium / Low	Low / High	Low
Strategy	Develop Product Portfolio	Secure Market Position	Capture Dominant Market Position	Redeploy Resources (Higher Return Areas)	Focus on Free Cash Flows
Resource Allocation	Invest	Invest	Invest	Maintain/Harvest	Harvest

Source: MMC International

- Nearly every major pharmaceutical development project is incorporating information on genetic variation and its effects on the safety and effectiveness of the candidate drug.
- Pharmacogenomic biomarkers are forecast to play an increasingly important role as patient selection and treatment stratification tools in drug development.
    - They will increasingly be required for product reimbursement.
- About 67% of Phase II and Phase III Products in the pharmaceuticals development pipeline have a biomarker for a genetic test.
- Over 1,300 genetic tests exist that signal susceptibility to a wide range of medical conditions.

Biomarkers is an emerging market that is forecast to grow exponentially.

The utilization of biomarkers, an emerging market, will grow exponentially, over the next ten years, to manage drug therapy, disease management, and in drug discovery. Biomarkers are measurements that provide information regarding a disease state or biological state that can be instrumental in disease management and drug discovery. There are five categories of biomarkers:

1. response,
2. efficacy,
3. toxicity,
4. dosing, and
5. screening/prognostic.

In 2010, there were over 200 product labels that either recommend genetic testing or point to the influence of genetic variation on drug response or safety.

Pharmacogenomic Testing Required On Product Label		
Therapy	**BioMarker/Test**	**Indication(s)**
Herceptin® (trastuzumab)	HER-2/neu receptor	Breast cancer
Tykerb® (lapatinib)	HER-2/neu receptor	Breast cancer
Erbitux® (cetuximab)	EGFR expression	Colon Cancer
Gefi tinib	EGFR expression	Colon Cancer
Vectibix® (panitumab)	EGFR expression	Colon Cancer
Gleevec® (imatinib mesylate)	BCR-ABL	Leukemia
Dasatinib	Philadelphia Chromosome	Leukemia
Selzentry® (maraviroc)	CCR5 receptor (1)	HIV

Pharmacogenomic Testing Recommended On Label		
Therapy	**BioMarker/Test**	**Indication(s)**
Coumadin® (warfarin)	CYP2C9	Cardiovascular
Coumadin® (warfarin)	VKORC1	Cardiovascular
Coumadin® (warfarin)	PGx PredictTM: Warfarin	Cardiovascular
Atorvastatin	LDLR	Cardiovascular
Camptosar® (irinotecan)	UGTIA1	Colon Cancer
Tegretol (carbamazepine)	HLA-B*1502	Epilepsy Bipolar Disorder
Ziagen® (abacavir)	HLA-B*5701	HIV
Purinethol® (mercaptopurine)	TPMT	Leukemia
Thioguanine	TPMT	Leukemia
Azathioprine	TPMT	Leukemia
Elitek® (rasburicase)	G6PD defi ciency	Multiple Cancers

Sources: U.S. FDA Table of Valid Genomic Biomarkers in the Context of Approved Drug Labels, accessed October 8, 2010, http://www.fda.gov/Drugs/ScienceResearch/ResearchAreas/Pharmacogenetics/ucm083378.htm and MMC International.

Biomarkers

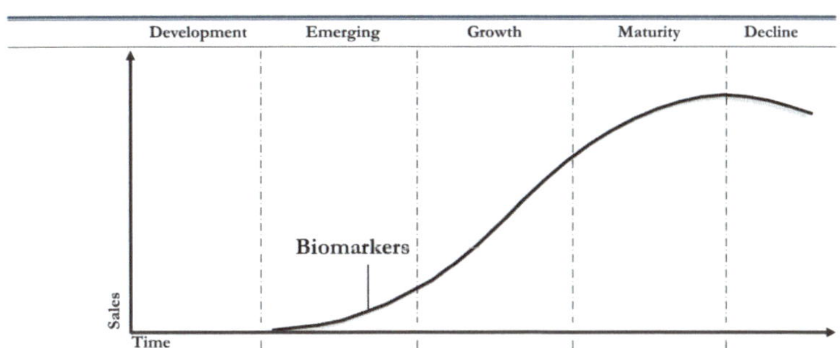

	Development	Emerging	Growth	Maturity	Decline
Risk	Medium	High / Medium	Medium / Low	Low / High	Low
Strategy	Develop Product Portfolio	Secure Market Position	Capture Dominant Market Position	Redeploy Resources (Higher Return Areas)	Focus on Free Cash Flows
Resource Allocation	Invest	Invest	Invest	Maintain/Harvest	Harvest

Source: MMC International.

Cybernetics, devices connectivity and medical "APPs" are rapidly emerging markets.

Cybernetics, provider, patients, medical information, and devices connectivity and medical "APPs" are rapidly emerging technologies/markets. They will transform how medicine is practiced, information is disseminated, and patients are diagnosed, treated and managed.

Cybernetics Physician Assistant

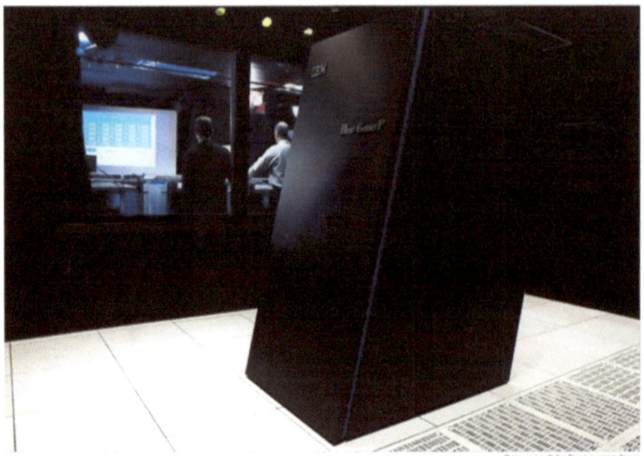

Cybernetics, Medical Apps and Connectivity Lifecycle

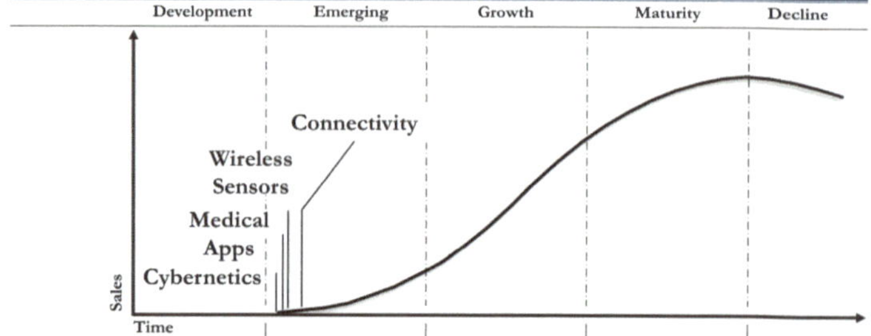

	Development	Emerging	Growth	Maturity	Decline
Risk	Medium	High / Medium	Medium / Low	Low / High	Low
Strategy	Develop Product Portfolio	Secure Market Position	Capture Dominant Market Position	Redeploy Resources (Higher Return Areas)	Focus on Free Cash Flows
Resource Allocation	Invest	Invest	Invest	Maintain/Harvest	Harvest

Source: MMC International.

The leading company in cybernetics is IBM. A leading company in medical instrument connectivity is Texas Instruments.

Connectivity and Medical APPs

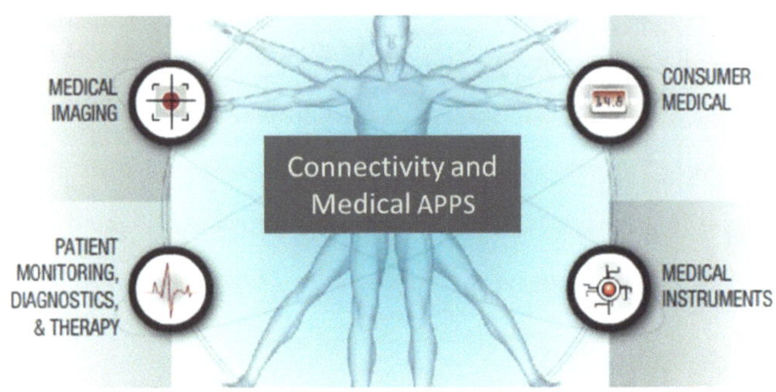

Automated External Defibrillator
Blood Gas Analyzer: Portable
Blood Pressure Monitor
CPAP Machine
CT Scanner
Confocal Microscopy
Dialysis Machine

ECG Electrocardiogram
Endoscope
Infusion Pump
Magnetic Resonance Imaging
Medical Meters: Portable
Patient Monitoring
Pulse Oximetry

Stethoscope: Digital
Telehealth Aggregation Manager
Telehealth Aggregation Manager with Video Output
Ultrasound System
Ultrasound System: Portable
Ventilator
X-ray: Medical/Dental

Smartphones plus Medical APPs and wireless sensors will be utilized to monitor patients on a real time basis, communicate data with care givers, and to check medical information, etc.

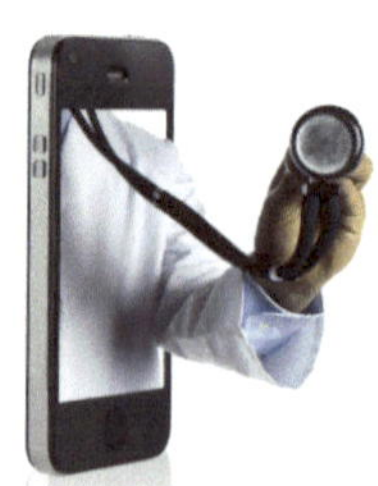

- In 2010, 85% of adult Americans had cell phones.
  - 15% used their cell phone to look for health information.
- 72% of American doctors owned smartphones.
- 86% of MDs, in a September 2010 PwC survey indicated they wanted mobile Electronic Medical Record access.

The first Cybernetic Physician Assistant application will go online by IBM for WellPoint in 2012.

The launch of IBM's Watson Cybernetics Physician Assistant technology in 2012 will begin the fundamental transformation (which will be implemented at an accelerating pace over the next ten years) of: 1) physicians/healthcare professionals training, 2), how diseases are defined, diagnosed, treated and managed, and 3) how medicine is practiced. Cybernetics will speed the adoption of new treatments/technology.

On February 17, 2011, I.B.M. executives said they planned to announce that it will collaborate with Columbia University and the University of Maryland to create a physician's assistant service that will allow doctors to query a cybernetic assistant. The company also plans to work with Nuance Communications Inc. to add voice recognition to the physician's assistant, possibly making the service available in as little as 18 months.

"I have been in medical education for 40 years and we're still a very memory-based curriculum," said Dr. Herbert Chase, a professor of clinical medicine at Columbia University who is working with I.B.M. on the physician's assistant. "The power of Watson-like tools will cause us to reconsider what it is we want students to do."

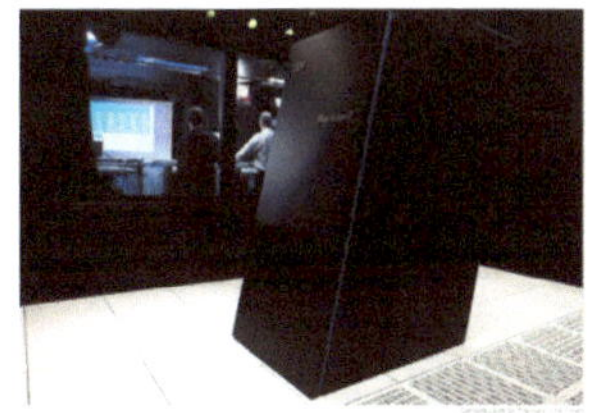

Launch in 2012 of the first cybernetics physician assistant service.

The first cybernetics physician assistant service (developed by IBM and named Watson) deployment is expected in 2012 when WellPoint nurses, who manage complex patient cases and review treatment requests from medical providers, begin using the system. Then, WellPoint, plans to roll out the technology to a small number of oncology practices, which would likely allow doctors to access it through their own computer systems or tablets. WellPoint hopes the service will improve quality of care, which it believes could lower costs.

WellPoint ultimately wants to provide the Watson service more broadly to physicians who treat complicated chronic conditions, and they hope to create an application that could be accessed directly by patients seeking health information.

Launch of new healthcare content and predictive analytics solution.

On October 27, 2011, IBM announced that by combining IBM's Watson technology with industry solutions offerings, Seton Healthcare Family (the top ranked healthcare system in Texas) intends to focus Watson's new content and predictive analytics solution on the root causes of hospital readmissions, and ways it can decrease preventable multiple hospital visits.

Seton Healthcare Family plans on using the Watson technology to leverage natural language to mine through tons of medical information, and "go far beyond traditional search and analysis of unstructured data," connecting previously unconnected information or helping doctors detect medical trends that would normally take long hours of paperwork to determine. According to IBM, if a business already is using IBM's Health Integration Framework solutions, dropping in Watson is an easy add-on. If a healthcare facility wants to deploy Watson, it will need one of IBM's Power Systems.

This emerging technology will redefine how healthcare is practiced in the future.

The emerging Medical APPS market will transform how patients are diagnosed, monitored and managed.

Medical APPs are an emerging market. In January 2010, there were over 1,700 iPhone medical APPS that had been downloaded by more than one million users to help monitor heart rates, manage diabetes, record exercise schedules, and link with larger computer systems for managing health records. Medical Apps, which are forecast to become a $2 billion market, can be developed for numerous types of processes including education, health management, data management, health information, to monitor certain values real time and trended (e.g., heart rates, glucose levels, etc.), manage diseases (e.g., diabetes), record exercise schedules, communicate with providers or patients, and SYNC with cars and link with larger computer systems for managing health records.

- 3D Medical Animation Videos
- Radiology Assistant – Medical Imaging and Radiology Reference and Education
- iMeds Medication Reference
- How to Avoid a Medication Mistake
- Medical Encyclopedia
- Concise Medical Dictionary (Oxford)
- Medical Spanish with Audio
- Family Medical History
- Medical Calculator
- Medication Tracker
- Medical Devices
- Medical Lab Tests
- Med Tracker – Drugs, Medications and Prescriptions
- Diabetes Mellitus – ipocketcards
- Diabetes Diary
- Diabetes Calculator

Sample Rx Company APPS

- Ichemo Diary by Merck & Co.
- Advanced Cardiovascular Life Support
- Care Connect by Johnson & Johnson
- Sleep Tracker for Tylenol PM by McNeil (Johnson & Johnson)

New iPhone Health APP Launch Trends
July 2008 to December 2009

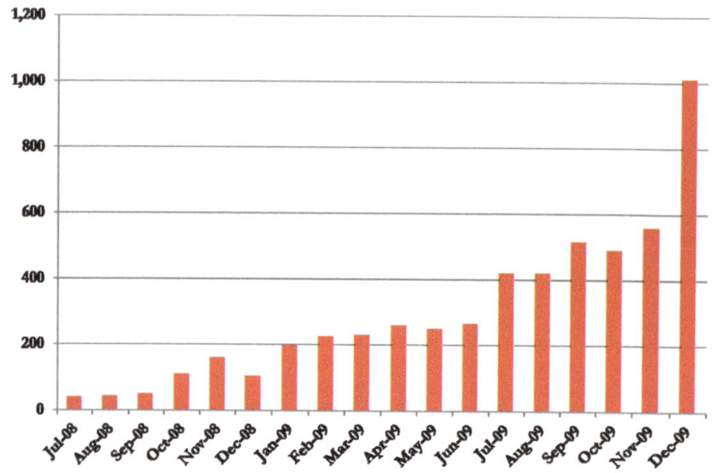

Source: vfluence, It Starts Online, January 2010.

In May 2011, The FDA's Center for Devices and Radiological Health stated it planned to issue guidelines on mobile medical applications in 2011. The FDA is concerned with issues of efficacy and safety as the development and usage of mobile medical apps gains momentum. Device and pharmaceutical companies have, are, and will develop proprietary APPs to assist in all aspects of product support, training, disease and patient management and marketing. The central component for managing individual health will become the smart phone.

3 INNOVATIONS

Innovations Will Fundamentally Transform U.S. Healthcare

Innovation in applying technologies, financial arrangements/incentives, standards, service offerings, networks, and/or organizational structures, etc. will effect all aspects of the U.S. healthcare industry between 2012 and 2020. They are evolving to redefine how products/services are reimbursed and where and how and by whom patients are screened, diagnosed, treated, managed and monitored, and treatments are classified/coded.

Implementation of ICD-10 will transform how diseases are classified, diagnosed, treated and managed.

The mandatory switch to ICD-10 diagnosis and procedures codes by October 2013, will unleash an increasing amount of data leading to better disease/condition management – and outcomes evaluations. On average, codes expand ICD-9 diagnosis and procedures codes by a factor of 8. ICD-10 coding, the personal genome incorporated into EHRs, and the ability to do mega data analysis will begin the fundamental transformation of how diseases are classified, diagnosed, treated and managed in the future.

Data structures will change significantly, as the number of new ICD-10 codes has increased dramatically.

Increase in codes as a result of clinical modifications, example of closed fracture of clavicle.

On average, codes expand by a factor of 8. Some codes expand less than 8 times and some as much as 144 times.

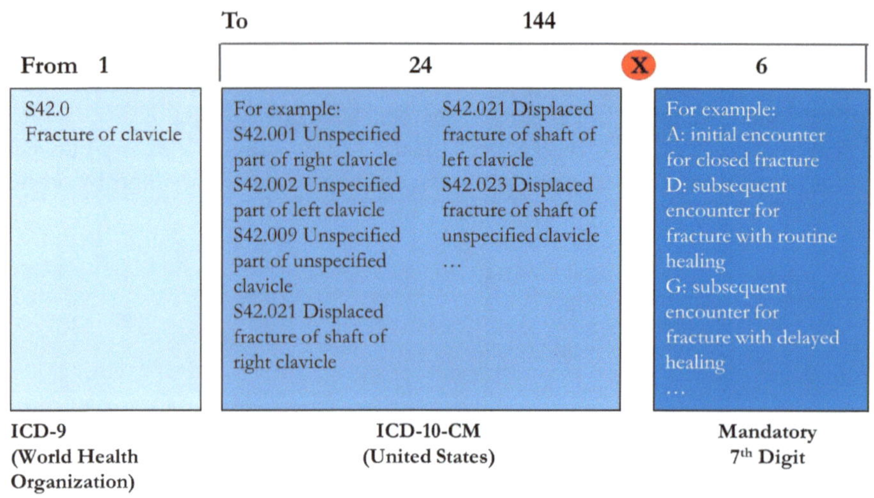

Source: Blue Cross and Blue Shield Association media briefing on moving to ICD-10, Sept 4, 2008; Centers for Medicare and Medicaid Services.

ICD-10

- The modern data format documenting diagnosis and procedure codes—ICD-10—was released by the United Nations (UN) World Health Organization in 1994.
    - Many developed countries, including Canada, Germany, and the United Kingdom, already use it.
- Payer compliance (and de-facto provider compliance) with the ICD-10 standard is mandatory by October 2013 and will be essential to exchange standardized data.
    - Failure to meet this date could result in significant penalties.
- ICD-10 expands the available number of ICD-9 medical codes by a factor of eight.
    - This change will enable a much more detailed description of diagnoses and treatments.
    - It will result in a tremendous growth in documentation of the medical details of diagnosis and treatment.
- ICD-10 will substantively influence a payer's medical management, network contracting, claims processing, customer service, actuarial, underwriting, and business intelligence functions.

ACOs are examples of care organizational models designed to improve care while reducing costs.

There are a myriad of efforts ongoing to organize patient care to improve outcomes while decreasing costs and maximizing provider profitability. The objective is to shift providers focus away from procedures to preventative care and wellness. Accountable Care Organizations (ACO) is a payment model incentivized in the PPACA legislation. ACOs are accountable for 100% of the expenditures and care for a defined population of patients.

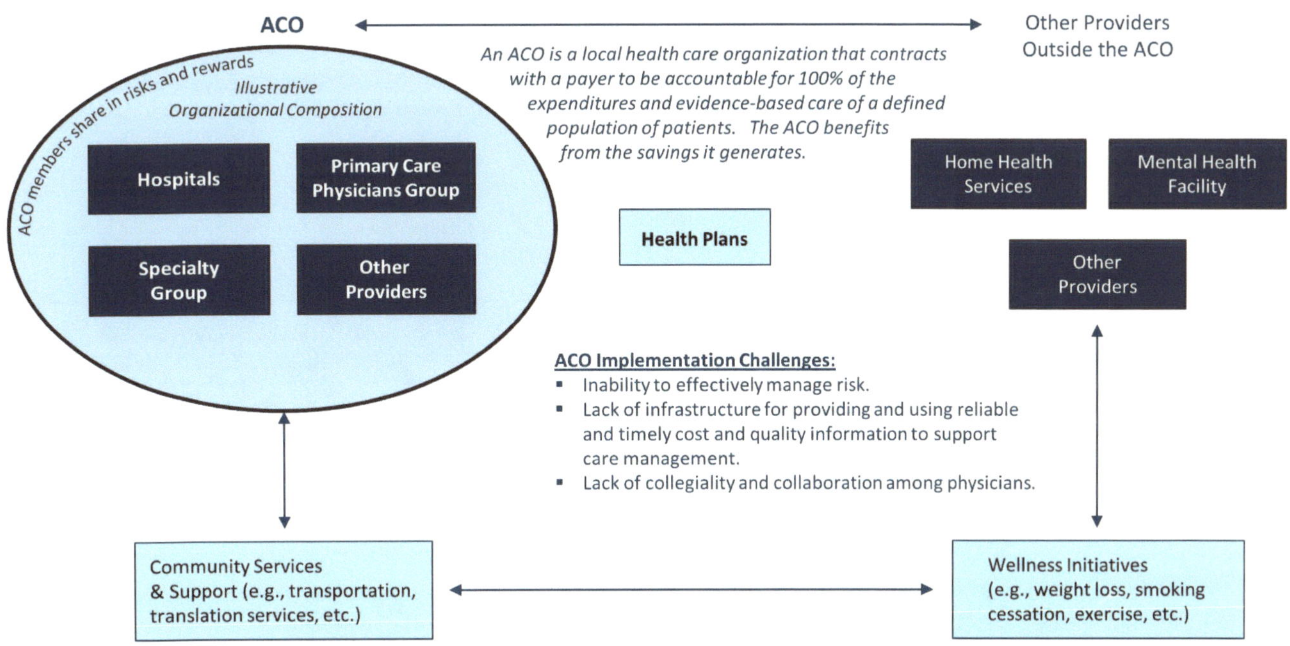

Sources: MMC International and Pricewaterhouse Coopers LLP Health Research Institute, September 2009 presentation.

ACOs are modeled after Mayo Clinic, Geisinger and Intermountain Healthcare, etc.

ACOs integrate local physicians with other members of the healthcare system and reward them for controlling costs and improving quality. The ACO concept is modeled after the Mayo Clinic, Geisinger and Intermountain Healthcare, etc.

Accountable Care Organizations

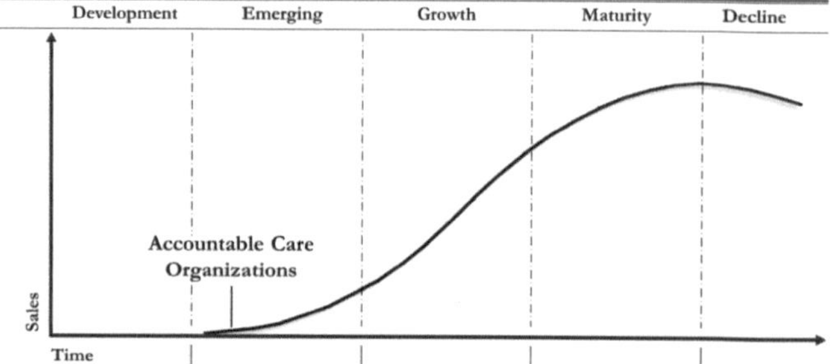

	Development	Emerging	Growth	Maturity	Decline
Risk	Medium	High / Medium	Medium / Low	Low / High	Low
Strategy	Develop Product Portfolio	Secure Market Position	Capture Dominant Market Position	Redeploy Resources (Higher Return Areas)	Focus on Free Cash Flows
Resource Allocation	Invest	Invest	Invest	Maintain/Harvest	Harvest

Source: MMC International.

- An ACO's innovation lies in the flexibility of their structure, payments and risk assumption.
  - They are not radically different from Health Maintenance Organizations (HMOs), physician-hospital organizations (PHOs) and independent practice associations (IPAs).
    - Unlike HMOs, PHOs and IPAs, ACOs rely on providers to review their own work and set standards rather than payers.
    - Additionally, by taking advantage of existing communities, rather than consolidating physician groups with hospitals as was done in the '90s, the resulting ACO would be a more harmonious construct.
  - They are similar to physicians in integrated healthcare delivery systems, such as the Mayo Clinic, Geisinger and Intermountain Healthcare.

- Paying for performance (P4P) is not novel. However, ACOs, rather than being held to a national benchmark derived from aggregate data, will be rewarded for achieving gains against its own baseline.
    - This will help control national spending while taking into account the wide variation in regional populations, practices and resulting spending.
- An Accountable Care Organization (ACO) may include primary care physicians, specialists and, typically, hospitals, that work together to provide evidence-based care in a coordinated model.
- The three major ACO functions are:
  - organization of all activities and accountability at the local level
  - measurement of longitudinal outcomes and costs
  - distribution of cost savings to ACO members.
- ACO physicians are accountable for the outcomes and expenditures of their assigned population and are tasked with collaboratively improving care to reach cost and quality targets set by the payer.
- A variety of federal, regional, state and academic hospital initiatives are investigating how to implement ACOs. The ACO pilots are being enabled by the exponential growth, decreasing costs, increasing ease of use, connectivity, and financial incentives to implement healthcare IT systems.

Under PPACA, ACOs will share savings realized by the Medicare program in each locality.

PPACA includes a Medicare pilot ACO program which shares savings realized by the Medicare program in each locality. The potential to share in billions in savings is and will serve to stimulate formation of ACOs through 2020.

- The PPACA ACO Medicare pilot program aims to explore optimal ACO structures and processes.
- Various provider organizations are eligible to become an ACO, including physician group practices, physician independent practice networks, partnerships between hospitals and physicians, and hospitals employing physicians.
    - A hospital is not a required component.
- The minimum requirements to be an ACO include:
    - shared governance
    - accountability for quality, costs and care
    - a clinical and administrative management structure
    - a primary care base sufficient to handle at least 5,000 Medicare beneficiaries.
- ACOs are required to have a formal legal structure to receive and distribute payments, and are eligible to receive a percentage of the annual shared savings.
- The U.S. Health and Human Services secretary is to set the annual threshold for eligible shared payments.
- The Medicare shared savings agreement is to be for not less than three years.
    - Any shared savings achieved are to be split between the Medicare program and the ACO.

Note: California's experience with ACOs may help predict whether accountable care organizations will work under the PPACA. "In California, many providers have been working in ACOs for decades, and they say they can work well--although there are pitfalls and limitations." Currently, around "half of insured Californians receive their care through some type of ACO." California's experience demonstrates that "aligning incentives and strong leadership are more important than the actual institutions;" that "varied payment mechanisms, instead of a one-size-fits-all approach, such as capitation" are important; and that "ACOs must not be fixed to only one insurance type." A pressing question is whether care coordination can "work in a PPO environment where consumer choice reigns...Pilot projects are under way in California that seek to collaborate among providers and payers across business lines." (Modern Healthcare, by Vesely, November 1, 2010).

ACOs will herald a period of provider innovation and consolidation not seen since the 1980s.

There is a high level of interest in ACOs. ACOs will herald a period of provider innovation and consolidation not seen since the HMO period of the 1980s. Consolidation will be driven by increased economies which will decrease costs and increase the profit sharing pool for providers. Consolidation does not mean ownership. Some consolidation will be contractual whereby certain back office operations are consolidated and a revenue sharing model is put into place. A lot of experimentation will take place over the next few years before dominant models emerge. The economies will be dictated on provider catchment area by catchment area. The key change will be a shift to objective health measures and care coordination and accountability. The change in thinking represents a cultural shift in how providers view their respective roles in patient wellness, care and management – as well as provider compensation.

Potential Accountable Care Organizations (ACO) Models And Their Characteristics

Provider Type	Ability to Provide or Manage Care Across Continuum	Ability to Plan Budgets and Resource Needs (Accept and manage non-FFS payment)	Provider Inclusiveness	Level of Performance Accountability
Independent practice association (IPA)	Low/Medium	Medium	High	Medium
Multispecialty Group	Medium/High	Medium	Low/Medium	Medium/High
Hospital Medical Staff Organization	Medium	Low/Medium	Medium	Low/Medium
Physician-Hospital Organization (PHO)	Medium/High	Medium/High	Low/Medium	Medium/High
Organized or Integrated Delivery Systems	Medium/High	Medium/High	Medium	Medium/High
Virtual approach-Extended Hospital Medical Staff	Medium	Low/Medium	High	Low

Sources: Chart adapted from What are Accountable Care Organizations?, Healthcare Economist, January 26, 2010.

As of December 1, 2011, there were 164 ACOs. This is before the PPACA required 2012 implementation of physician payment reforms in Medicare to enhance primary care services and encourage doctors to form "accountable care organizations" to improve quality and efficiency of care. Of the 164 "ACO entities" found in a study by Leavitt Partners, 99 were sponsored by hospital systems, 38 by physician groups and 27 by insurers. They were located in 41 states, though there were vast regional differences. Poor and rural regions were found to have little ACO growth.

The emerging PCMH model is expected to become the prevalent care cost savings innovation.

The emerging patient-centered medical home (PCMH), initially developed in 2006, is an innovative model of primary care delivery that promotes care coordination as a necessary replacement for volume-based incentives that limit primary care physicians' (PCP) effectiveness. The clinical and economic potential is promising. Work on developing an optimal model will persist through 2020. The PCMH is expected to become a prevalent care cost-savings innovation. It is enabled by information sharing through interoperable electronic health records (EHRs). It enhances coordination and connectivity between care teams. PPACA legislation calls for five major patient-centered medical home (PCMH) initiatives encompassing testing and evaluation, performance, financial incentives, quality measures, and implementation assistance.

PPACA Patient-centered Medical Home Initiatives

PPACA PCMH Initiative	Description
Innovation Center	The Center for Medicare and Medicaid Innovation will be testing and evaluating models that include medical homes as a way of addressing defined populations with either: 1) poor clinical outcomes, or 2) avoidable expenditures.
Health Plan Performance	Medical homes are identified as one performance indicator for health plans. Additionally, the state health insurance exchanges are designing incentives to encourage high-performance plans, including those with medical homes.
Chronic Medicaid Enrollee Care	Starting in 2011, the federal government will match state funds, up to 90 percent for two years, for states that provide options for Medicaid enrollees with chronic conditions to receive their care under a medical home model.
Community Care	To encourage the establishment of medical homes in community health systems, PPACA is providing grants to community care teams that organize themselves under the medical home model.
New Model for Training	In conjunction with the Agency for Health Research & Quality (AHRQ), PPACA creates the Primary Care Extension Program, which provides primary care training and implementation of medical home quality improvement and processes.

Patient-centered Medical Home

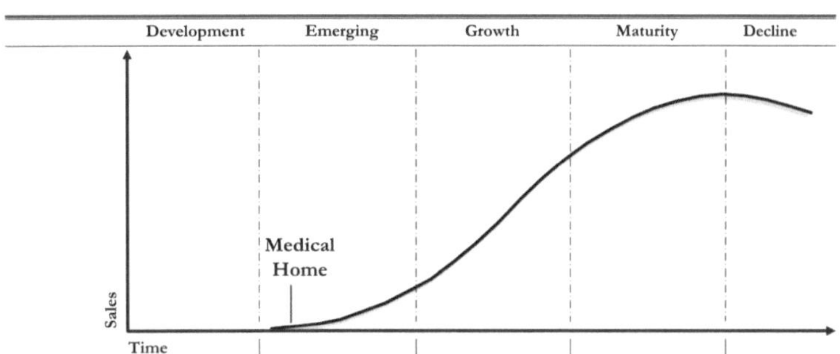

	Development	Emerging	Growth	Maturity	Decline
Risk	Medium	High / Medium	Medium / Low	Low / High	Low
Strategy	Develop Product Portfolio	Secure Market Position	Capture Dominant Market Position	Redeploy Resources (Higher Return Areas)	Focus on Free Cash Flows
Resource Allocation	Invest	Invest	Invest	Maintain/Harvest	Harvest

Source: MMC International.

The PCMH model saves money by delivering continuous patient-oriented primary care.

The goal of the PCMH is to deliver continuous, accessible, high-quality, patient-oriented primary care. Pilot programs have shown that PCMH improves patient care/outcomes while saving money. It has been widely touted by a number of medical associations, e.g., American Academy of Family Physicians (AAFP), American Academy of Pediatrics (AAP), American Osteopathic Association (AOA), American College of Physicians (ACP), as a means of reducing long-term healthcare costs associated with chronic diseases – from pediatric to the elderly.

The American Academy of Pediatrics (AAP) first introduced the medical home concept in 1967, and subsequently in 2006. In 2007, four associations, the American Academy of Family Physicians (AAFP), AAP, American Osteopathic Association (AOA) and the American College of Physicians (ACP) released the following Joint Principles of the Patient-centered Medical Home:

Summary of Joint Principles of the Patient-Centered Medical Home

Principle	Description
Personal physician	• Patients are assigned to a personal physician who provides "first contact, continuous and comprehensive care".
Physician-directed medical practice	• Personal physician leads all other health care providers in the patient's care.
"Whole person" orientation	• Personal physician is responsible for all of the patient's care, including acute, chronic, preventive and end-of-life care.
Integrated and coordinated care	• Care is coordinated across all facilities through health care technology.
Quality and safety	• Practice collaborates with patient and family to define a patient-centered care plan. • Practice uses evidence-based medicine and care pathways. • Practice performs continuous quality improvement by measuring and reporting performance metrics. • Patient feedback is incorporated into performance measurement. • Patients and families participate in practice quality improvement. • Information technology is a foundation of patient care, performance measurement, communication and patient education. • Practices are certified as patient-centered by non-governmental entities . • Physicians share in savings from reduced hospitalizations. • Physicians receive bonus payments for attaining predetermined quality metrics.
Enhanced access to care	• Patients can take advantage of open scheduling, expanded hours and new communication options with the physician practice.
Payments that recognize primary care added value	• Payments should reflect both physician and non-physician value and encompass payments for all services, including non-face-to-face visits and care management.

Medical Home Pilot Program Savings Per Patient

Pilot Program	# of Patients	Population	Incentives	Results (Savings)		
				Hospitalization Reduction (%)	ER Visit Reduction (%)	Total Savings Per Patient
Colorado Medical Home for Children	**10,781**	**Medicaid CHP+**	**Pay for Performance (P4P)**	**18%**	**N/A**	**$169-$530**
Community Care of North Carolina	**>1 Million**	**Medicaid**	**Per Member Per Month (PMPM) Payment**	**40%**	**16%**	**$516**
Geisinger (Provent-HealthNavigator)	**TBD**	**Medicare Advantage**	**P4P; PMPM Payment; Shared Savings**	**15%**	**N/A**	**N/A**
Group Health Cooperative	**9,200**	**All**	**TBD**	**11%**	**29%**	**71%**
Intermountain Health Care (Care Management Plus)	**4,700**	**Chronic Disease**	**P4P**	**4.8%-19.2%**	**0%-7.3%**	**$640**
MeritCare Health System and Blue Cross Blue Shield of North Dakota	**192**	**Diabetes**	**PMPM Payment; Shared Savings**	**6%**	**24%**	**$530**
Vermont BluePrint for Health	**60,000**	**All**	**PMPM Payment**	**11%**	**12%**	**$215**

Sources: Excerpted from Fields D., Leshen E., and Patel K. "Driving gains and cost savings through adoption of medical homes", Health Affairs, May 2010; 29(5): 819-826. Appendix Exhibit 1; and Deloitte.

Retail clinics are an emerging market which is expected to become profitable before 2020.

Retail clinics, which began to grow around 2000, are an emerging market. They are innovating regarding structure, services, locations, strategic alliances, and methods to become profitable. These issues are expected to be resolved between 2013 and 2020.

Retail Health Clinics

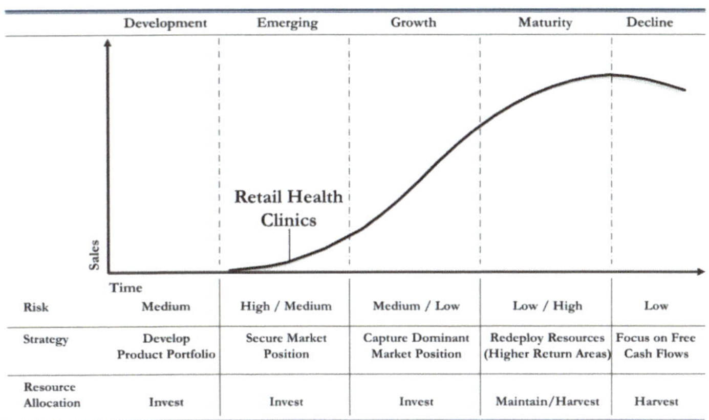

Source: MMC International

Retail Health Clinics

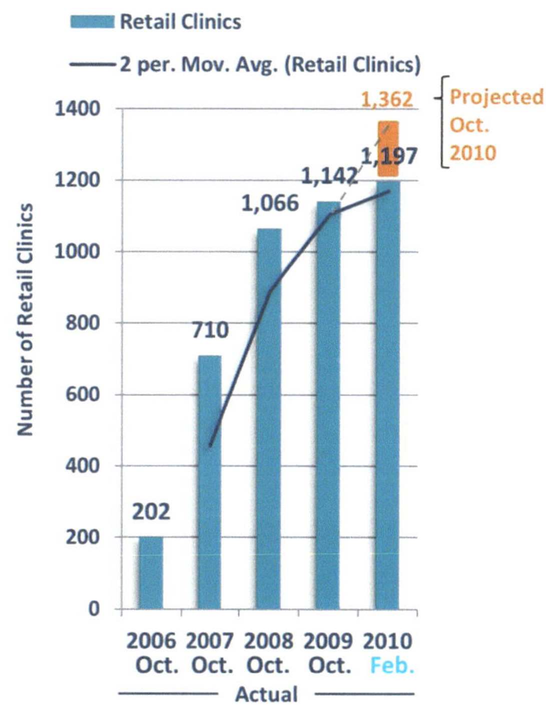

Sources: MMC International trend and Merchant Medicine statistics.

Retail Clinic Growth By Major Players

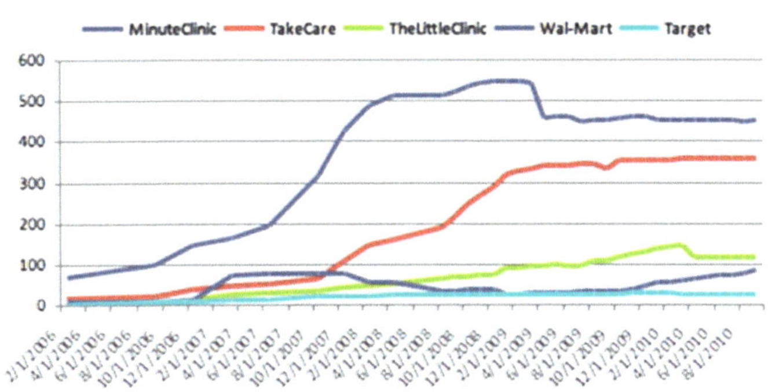

Sources: http://www.merchantmedicine.com/Home.cfm?view=Retail by Merchant Medicine

The structure of the Retail Clinics industry will be decided by development of a profitable business model.

The structure of the Retail Clinics market will be decided by the development of a profitable business model. Profitability appears to favor drug store chains, mass merchandiser and/or food stores with pharmacies, and hospitals/integrated delivery systems.

September 2009 RAND Study Findings

- Overall costs of care for episodes initiated at retail clinics were substantially lower than those of matched episodes initiated at physician offices and urgent care centers($110 vs. $166) , and emergency departments ($156 vs. $570).
- Prescription costs were similar in retail clinics, physician offices, and urgent care centers ($21, $21, and $22).
- Aggregate quality scores were similar (63.6%, 61.0%, and 62.6%).
- Patient's receipt of preventive care was also about the same (14.5%, 14.2%, and 13.7%).
- In emergency departments, average prescription costs were higher and aggregate quality scores were significantly lower than in other settings.

Source: Comparing Costs and Quality of Care at Retail Clinics With That of Other Medical Settings for 3 Common Illnesses by Ateev Mehrotra, MD; Hangsheng Liu, PhD; John L. Adams, PhD; Margaret C. Wang, PhD; Judith R. Lave, PhD; N. Marcus Thygeson, MD; Leif I. Solberg, MD; and Elizabeth A. McGlynn, PhD From RAND Health.

Retail Health Clinics Companies
August 2010

- AirportMD
- Alegent Health Quick Care
- Aspirus FastCare Clinic
- AtlantiCare /HealthRite
- Aurora QuickCare
- BDCH Fast Care
- Bellin Health FastCare
- Blessing FastCare
- Careworks Convenient Healthcare
- CHRISTUS Medical Group
- CMG CareToday
- Consumer Health Services, Inc.
- Cox Health Systems
- Curaquick Clinic
- CVS Caremark MinuteClinic
- DR Walk-In Medical Care
- Drexel Convenient Care Center
- ExpressCare Clinic
- Express Clinics, Inc.
- ExpressHEALTH Clinic
- Fairview Express Care Clinic
- Family Quick Care
- FHN FastCare
- Froedtert FastCare
- Gunderson Lutheran ExpressCare Clinic
- Harmony Pharmacy & Health Center
- HealthPartners HealthStation
- Heritage Valley ConvenientCare
- Intermountain ExpressCare
- Iowa Health Express Care
- Lindora Health Clinics
- Marquette General FastCare
- Mayo Express Care
- MediGo
- MediMin, Inc.
- MEDPOINT express
- Mercy Quick Care Clinic
- MeritCare FastTrack
- Meriter FastCare Clinics
- Monroe FastCare
- MultiCare Express
- NorthReach FastCare
- Northwest Health System
- NOW Medical Centers
- OMC FastCare
- Owensboro Medical Health System
- PPH expresscare
- Premier ExpressCare
- QuickHealth, Inc.
- RediClinic
- Roadside Medical Labs and Clinics
- Saint Alphonsus Express Care
- Solantic
- St. Luke's Q Care
- St. Nicholas Hospital FastCare
- SUPERVALU
- Sutter Express Care
- Target Clinic
- The AeroClinic
- The Little Clinic
- ThedaCare FastCare
- UW Watertown FastCare
- Valley Health Quick Care
- ValueCare Medical Clinic
- Walgreens Health and Wellness
- The Clinic at Walmart
- WellnessMart

Social networking is a transformational technology that will change information access and sharing.

Social networking in 2012 is what online access was just 20 years ago – a transformational change in how information is accessed and shared. It will transform health information sharing over the next ten years.

- About one-third of Americans who go online to research their health currently use social networks to find fellow patients and discuss their conditions.[1,2]
- 36 percent of social network users evaluate and leverage other consumers' knowledge before making healthcare decisions.[3]
- Social networks hold considerable potential value for healthcare organizations because they can be used to:
  – reach stakeholders
  – aggregate information
  – leverage collaboration.

2010 Social Network Examples

Network	Usage	Description
YouTube	>6.5 Billion Views	Video Postings
Facebook	>500 Million Registered Users, 30% in U.S., >50 Million Active Users	Recreational Peer-to-Peer Social Network
Twitter	>105 Million Registered Users, 51% in U.S.	
LinkedIn	>60 Million, 50% in U.S.	Professional Peer-to-Peer Networking
Yelp	>30 Million Visitors Per Month	Crowd Sourced Reviews of Local Businesses
MySpace	>57 Unique U.S. Users	Social Networking
Blogs	149.7 Million Blogs as of November 1, 2010 (BlogPost)	Web Journal Which Chronologically Presents Posts
Wikis	14.7 Million Views Per Hour	Collaborative Data Creation and Editing of a Number of Interlinked Web Pages
Forums and Discussion Boards	Approximately 50% of Americans That Use the Internet Use Peer-to-Peer Social Networking	Special Interest Social Networks

1 Manhattan Research's Cybercitizen Health v9.0.
2 Noah Elkin, "How America Searches: Health and Wellness," iCrossing, January 2008.
3 Jupiter Research, Online Health: Assessing the risks and opportunity of social and one-to-one media, 2007.
Sources: Internet searches conducted by MMC International and company annual reports and presentations.

Other innovations through 2020 will transform patient diagnosis, treatment and management.

A myriad of other innovations, e.g., cloud computing, telemedicine, connected home care, Biophotonics, smart Apps, etc., will progress over the next ten years and will transform how and where patients are diagnosed, treated, monitored, and managed. Each will incorporate a number of new and emerging technologies to develop a service to cost-effectively change provider practices. The only known is that they will be developed and that a number of them will appear for the first time sometime between 2012 and 2020. Some will be computer/wi-fi enabled while others will be scientific/device/process enhancements.

Computer/Wi-Fi/Internet Enabled

- ***Cloud computing*** – enabling users (all size corporations as well as consumers and patients) to take advantage of sophisticated computing capabilities, data warehousing, and collaborative working venues without the requirement of IT staffs.

- ***Telemedicine*** - videoconferencing, virtual or online care on demand, virtual or online medical training, remote patient monitoring, telediagnostics, home telehealth, mobile health, clinical mobility, aging in place, health information exchanges, electronic health records, medical call centers, outsourced clinical services, etc.

- ***Connected home care*** (enabling care at home) - in-home technologies can increase medication adherence, provide intervention required alerts and improve chronic condition management.

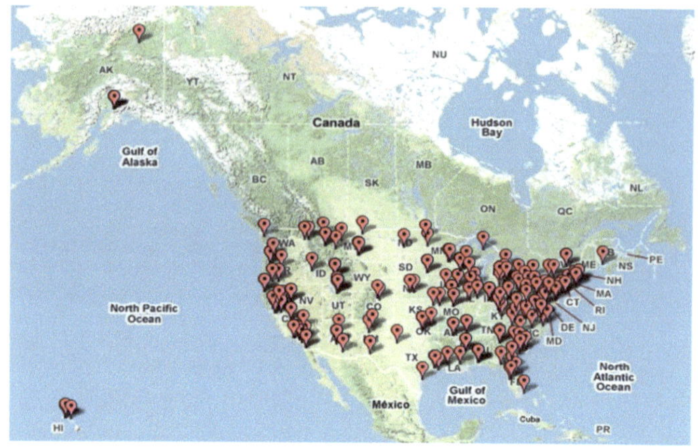

According to the American Telemedicine Association (ATA), there were approximately 200 medical center-based telemedicine networks operating in the United States in 2010 – linking over 2,500 institutions nationwide. The type of services provided as well as the network configuration varies widely. These 2,500 networks do not include many other categories of telemedicine such as medical call centers, home telehealth, remote monitoring or outsourced clinical services.

- ***Biophotonics/Smart Apps*** - health monitoring using a cell phone, personal health record on personal cell phones, integration of devices and blood analysis with remote monitoring (e.g., an integrated pump with a continuous blood glucose monitor in communication with a patient monitoring service/disease management service), tracking of disease progression, e.g., malaria and HIV using cell phone based blood analysis (e.g., using shadow imaging blood analysis).

These innovations represent new product, product differentiation and value packaging opportunities.

These innovations, e.g., surgical and mechanical interventions, stem cells, regenerative medicine, etc., will effect pharmaceutical prescribing, persistence and compliance. They will open opportunities for product differentiation and value-added packaging. All are in the emerging stages of their Lifecycles.

Scientific/Device/Process Advancements

- ***Surgical and mechanical interventions*** – will be developed using new and existing technologies. These advances, like bronchial thermoplasty, may change the course of a disease or minimize or eliminate symptoms – thereby decreasing the demand for certain medications.

- ***Stem cells*** – an estimated $300 million business in 2010, is forecast to grow exponentially from 2011 through 2020. It has the potential to transform therapy for a myriad of traumatic, degenerative and autoimmune diseases – thereby effecting change for certain drug therapies.

- ***Regenerative medicine*** - At Wake Forest University, Dr. Anthony Atala has built, from the cell level up, 18 different types of tissue so far, including muscle tissue, whole organs and the pulsing heart valve of a sheep. In May 2008, fourteen large mammals were implanted with the neo-bladder construct and within six months, structure and pharmacological characteristics of the neo-bladder were similar to the native bladder, with no evidence of abnormal tissue development, immune response or evidence of systemic response to the neo-bladder regeneration. Results suggest that the new organ had successfully and safely regenerated.

Computer/Wi-Fi/Internet Enabled

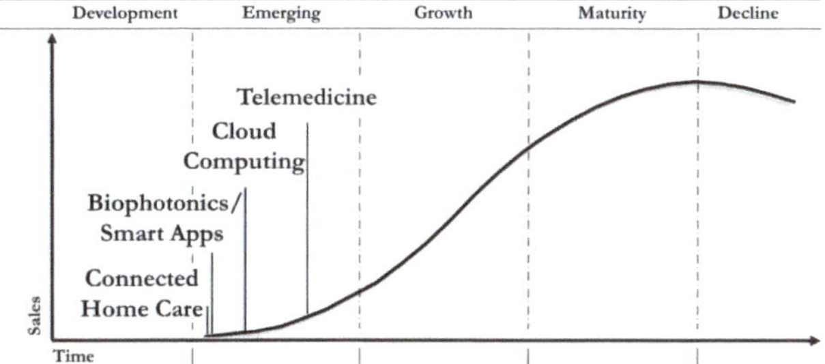

	Development	Emerging	Growth	Maturity	Decline
Risk	Medium	High / Medium	Medium / Low	Low / High	Low
Strategy	Develop Product Portfolio	Secure Market Position	Capture Dominant Market Position	Redeploy Resources (Higher Return Areas)	Focus on Free Cash Flows
Resource Allocation	Invest	Invest	Invest	Maintain/Harvest	Harvest

Source: MMC International.

Scientific/Device/Process Advancements

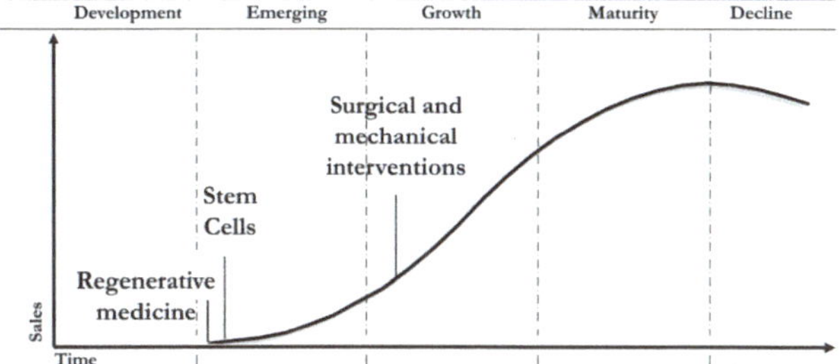

	Development	Emerging	Growth	Maturity	Decline
Risk	Medium	High / Medium	Medium / Low	Low / High	Low
Strategy	Develop Product Portfolio	Secure Market Position	Capture Dominant Market Position	Redeploy Resources (Higher Return Areas)	Focus on Free Cash Flows
Resource Allocation	Invest	Invest	Invest	Maintain/Harvest	Harvest

Source: MMC International.

4 THE U.S. HAS TO CONTAIN HEALTHCARE COSTS

Rising healthcare costs, if not corrected, will destroy the "American Dream" and the U.S. middle class.

Between 1999 and 2009, the typical median-income American family of four grew by about $22,920, from $76,200 in 1999 to $99,120 in 2009 in 2009 constant dollars. Increases in the prices of consumer goods and non-healthcare taxes absorbed 52 percent of the increase. Most of the rest was consumed by higher healthcare co-pays, deductibles, drug and medical supplies costs. This left the average American family with only $1,140 more per year in 2009 versus 1999, $95 more per month. If taxes had kept pace with the growth in federal healthcare spending for Medicare, Medicaid and other public health programs during the same period, the typical American family would have paid an additional $4,680 in taxes in 2009. This would have reduced average family disposable income by $3,540 in 2009 versus 1999 – significantly decreasing U.S. personal disposable income and American's quality of life. Historically, the cost of care has been obscured for American families. However, employees are facing increases in cost-sharing and out-of-pocket expenses which is making American's sensitive to the true cost of healthcare. The steep decline in access and affordability of healthcare, if not corrected, will destroy the "American Dream" and the U.S. middle class.

Real Average Family Income Declined $3,450, 4.6 Percent, Between 1999 and 2009
If Uncorrected, The Quality Of Life In The United States Will Decline

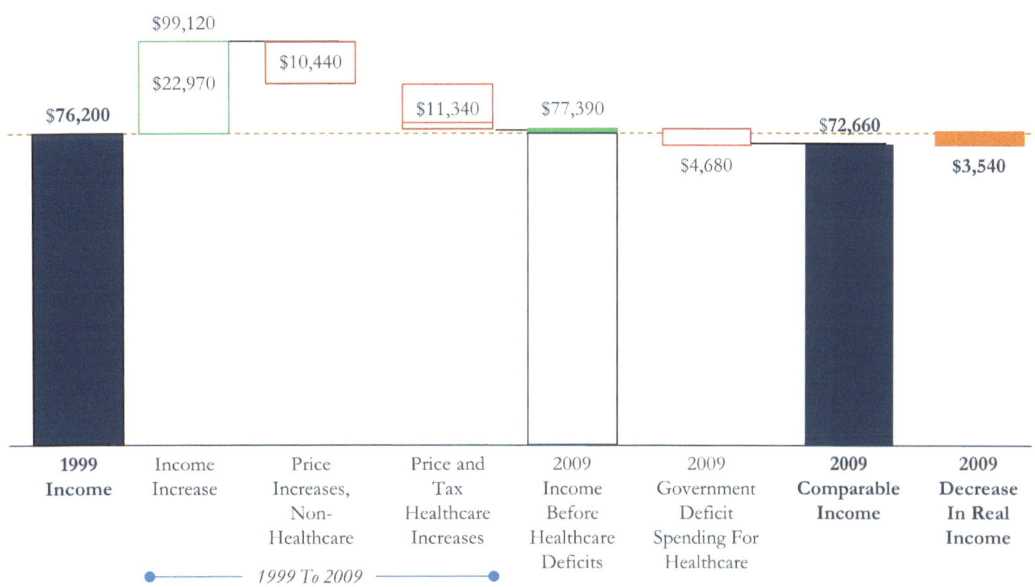

Note: No single data source can provide a complete picture of an average family's finances. The Rand study utilized, in MMC's opinion, reasonable assumptions in preparing their income estimates. Income is in constant 2009 dollars. Net health insurance benefits are factored in net of tax benefits. Annual incomes include employer-paid health insurance premium contributions as they more accurately represent changes in healthcare costs and contributions over time.
Sources: MMC International and Auerbach DI and Kellermann AL, "A Decade of Healthcare Cost Growth Has Wiped Out Real Income Gains for an Average U.S. Family," Health Affairs, Vol. 30, No. 9, September 2011. David I. Auerbach is a health economist at RAND in Boston, Massachusetts and Arthur L. Kellermann is vice president and director of RAND Health, in Santa Monica, California.

U.S. per capita health expenditures are forecast to grow at 5.2 percent annually through 2020.

Despite efforts to control healthcare costs, U.S. per capita health expenditures are forecast to grow from $8,047 in 2009 to $14,101 in 2020, at 5.2 percent annually.

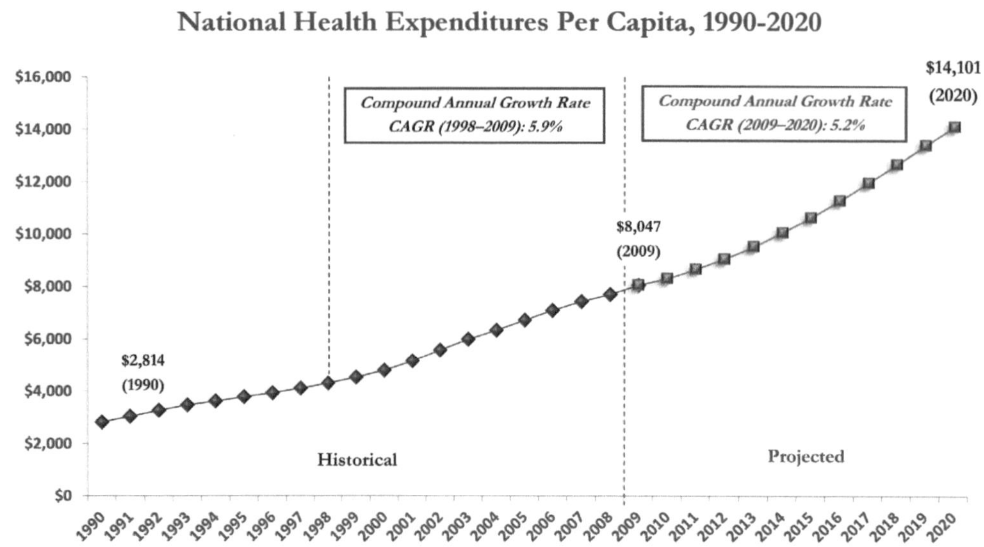

Sources: Centers for Medicare and Medicaid Services, Office of the Actuary, National Health Statistics Group, at http://www.cms.hhs.gov/NationalHealthExpendData/ (Historical data from NHE summary including share of GDP, CY 1960-2008, file nhegdp08.zip; Projected data from NHE Projections 2009-2019, Forecast summary and selected tables, file proj2009.pdf). 2020 Projection by MMC International.

The increasing cost of healthcare, if uncorrected, will compromise America's ability to compete.

The United States spends >5 percent more of its GDP on healthcare (HC) than any of the other 33 Organization for Economic Cooperation and Development (OECD) countries. Forecasted increases in healthcare (HC) expenditures and their share of GDP will continue pressure on all healthcare industry participants and federal and state legislatures to decrease healthcare costs while improving the quality of care. If uncorrected, healthcare costs will compromise America's ability to compete as the cost of healthcare is a cost component in every product sold.

Healthcare Expenditures as a % of GDP In OECD Countries In 2007

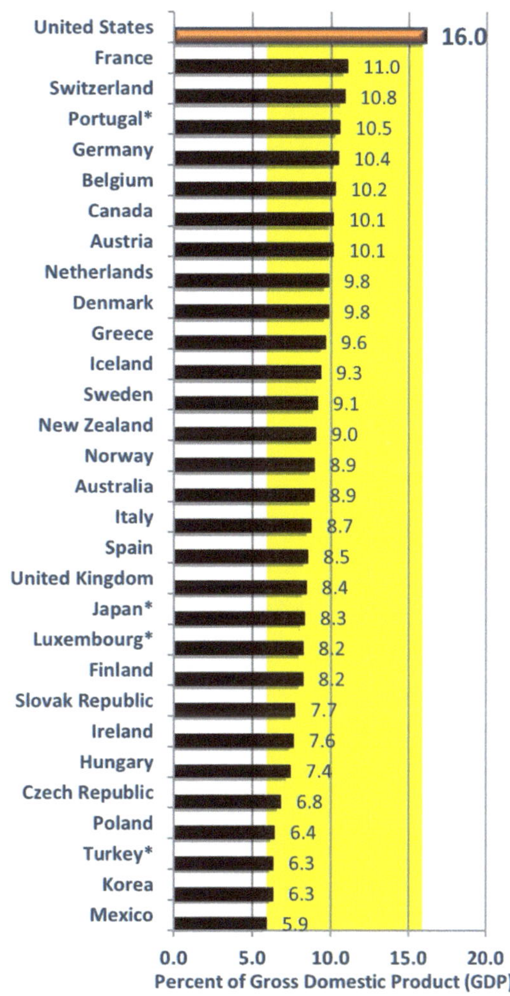

***** = Estimated projection from prior 10 years of data.
OECD = Organization for Economic Cooperation and Development
Sources: OECD Health Data 2009 – Version: November 09 and MMC International analysis.

5 INCREASING DEMAND

The aging population will drive up U.S. healthcare demand and utilization.

The growing ≥65 aging U.S. population, with their increasing number of chronic conditions and increasing lifespans, will drive up healthcare costs and the demand for coordinated, outcomes-based, preventative healthcare. Fifty eight percent, 18.0 million (MM), of the 2010 to 2020 U.S. population growth of 31.2 million, will be in the ≥45 years age bracket – which utilizes more care. This is and will cause all payers, insurers, providers and consumers to look for innovative ways to contain costs.

Average 2007 U.S. Spending Per Person By Age Group	
Age (in years)	
<5	$1,761
5-17	1,245
18-24	1,452
25-44	2,360
45-64	5,474
65 or Older	9,357
Sex	
Male	$3,319
Female	4,139

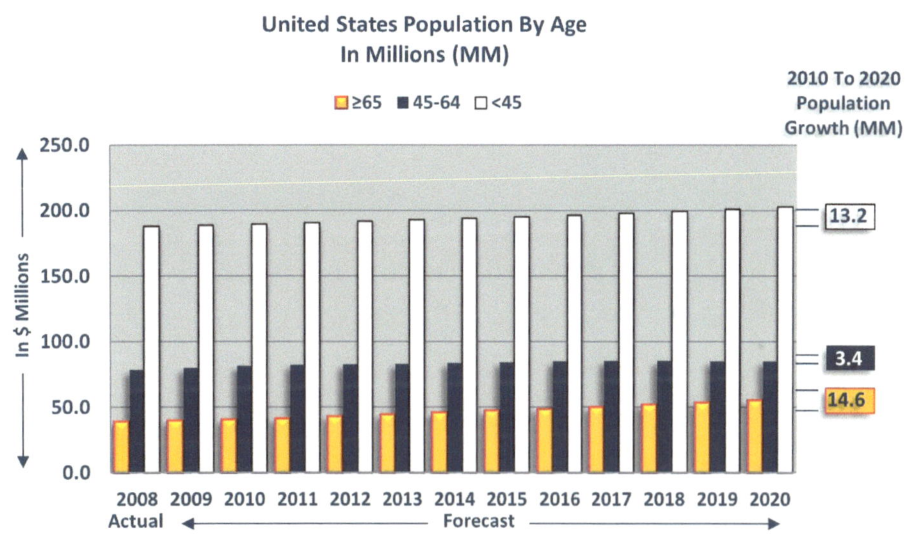

Sources: Average 2007 US Spending Per Person from Kaiser Family Foundation calculations using data from U.S. Department of Health and Human Services, Agency for Healthcare Research and Quality, Medical Expenditure Panel Survey (MEPS), 2007. Population statistics from: Population Division, U.S. Census Bureau Release date August 14, 2008, file 2008 National Population Projections. MMC International analysis.

6 THE OPPORTUNITY

Extraction of trillions of dollars in U.S. Healthcare inefficiencies by 2020 is an unprecedented opportunity.

U.S. Healthcare inefficiencies, if not addressed, will cost the U.S. $13.1 trillion dollars between 2011 and 2020. If five to seven percent of the inefficiencies are eliminated each year, on top of the changes that were already made in 2010, the U.S. would save in the neighborhood of $3.9 trillion between 2011 and 2020. Achieving these savings would maintain U.S. healthcare expenditures at or below 2009/2010 spending levels. Sharing the savings from extracting $13.1 trillion wasted healthcare expenditures is available under PPACA legislation. It is also rewarded by payers and providers who are competing for increased market share and shareholder returns. The overall opportunity is equivalent to about 10 percent of the U.S. GDP every year. The total potential 2011 to 2020 savings of $13.1 trillion almost equals the $14.7 2010 United States gross domestic product.

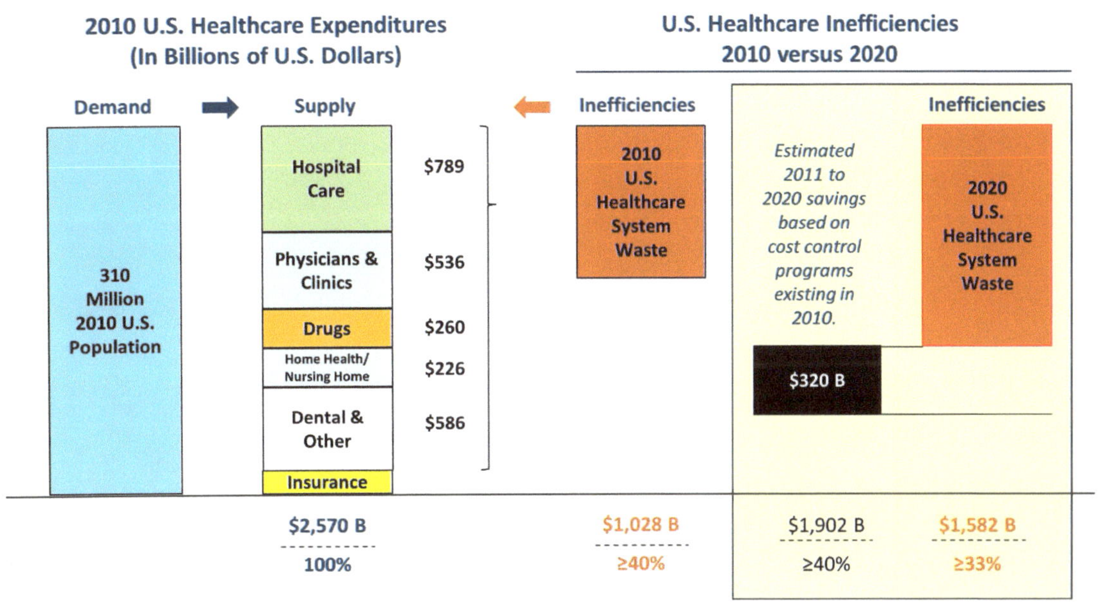

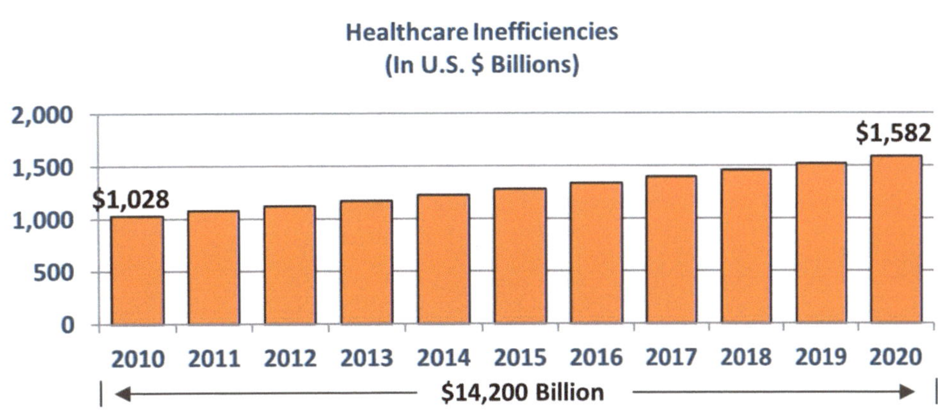

Sources: Centers for Medicare & Medicaid Services, Office of the Actuary and MMC International.

Implementation of new technologies and innovations are key to extracting U.S. healthcare inefficiencies.

Unlike other industries, U.S. healthcare is inefficient. It has been slow to implement information technology - contributing to duplicative care and the 17-year delay in universal adoption of best practices.

Doctors Use of Electronic Patient Medical Records

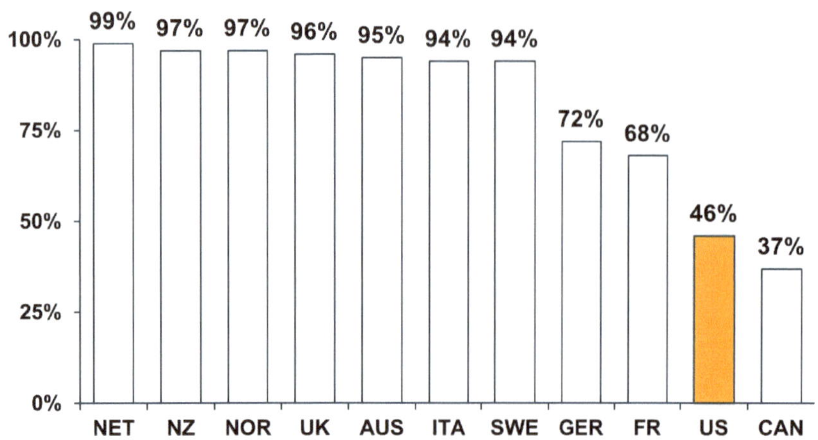

Note: Not including billing systems.
Source: C. Schoen, R. Osborn, M. M. Doty, D. Squires, J. Peugh, and S. Applebaum, "A Survey of Primary Care Physicians in 11 Countries, 2009: Perspectives on Care, Costs, and Experiences," *Health Affairs* Web Exclusive, Nov. 5, 2009, w1171–w1183.

The healthcare industry spends only 2% of gross revenues on health information technology (HIT), which is low compared to other information intensive industries such as finance, which spend upwards of 10%.

Sample of Select Functionalities and Their Level of Implementation in U.S. Non-Federal Hospitals

	Fully Implemented Across All Units
Electronic Clinical Documentation	
Medication Lists	45%
Nursing Assessments	36%
Physician Notes	12%
Problem Lists	27%
Results Viewing	
Diagnostic Test Images (e.g. EKG)	37%
Diagnostic Test Results (e.g. Echo)	52%
Lab Reports	77%
Radiology Images	69%
Radiology Reports	78%
Computerized Provider Order Entry	
Laboratory Tests	20%
Medications	17%

Source: Jha AK, DesRoches CM, Campbell EG, et al. "Use of Electronic Health Records in U.S. Hospitals." *New England Journal of Medicine*, 360(16):1628–1638, 2009.

Employing market forces to eliminate healthcare inefficiencies is key to eliminating U.S. healthcare waste.

U.S. healthcare legislation has fragmented care delivery and driven up healthcare costs through duplication of services, administration and infrastructure – while inconveniencing patients. The only way to reverse these inefficiencies is to eliminate or modify existing regulations and employ free market competition to correct these inefficiencies. How providers are compensated also needs to be addressed.

Fragmentation Of U.S. Healthcare

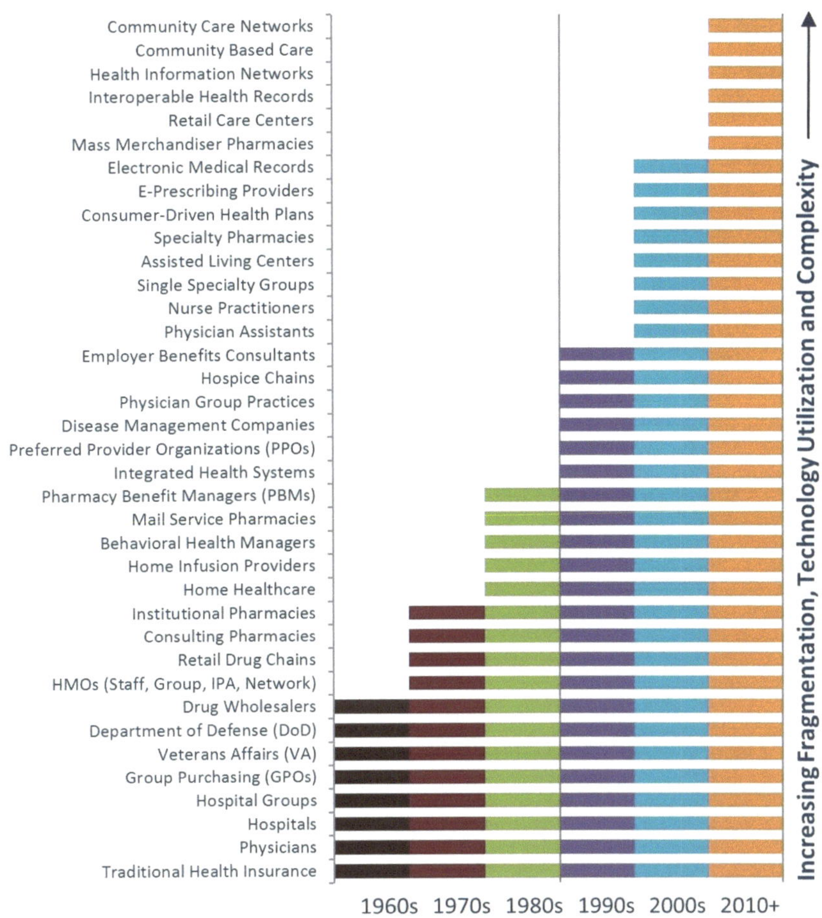

Source: MMC International.

Cost Duplication/Escalation

- Care Duplication
- Slower Implementation of Best Practices
- Administration
- Facilities
- Purchasing
- Patient Records
- Computer Systems
- Facility Certification
- Distribution Costs
- Shrinkage/Outdated Products
- Working Capital Costs
- Insurance Costs
- Reimbursement Costs
- Transportation Costs
- Equipment Costs
- Supplies Costs
- Lost Time (Patient)
- Lost Wages (Patient or Employer)
- Lost Productivity

Payers have to implement incentives that result in a desired outcome as a person or entity pursues their own self-interest. Paying for desired results is the only way U.S. healthcare will undo the damage that has been done.

7 LEGISLATIVE DRIVERS

The government's view of healthcare will drive legislation and implementing regulations.

It is important to understand what has prompted the government to act and how these viewpoints will influence implementation of regulations and guidelines. In turn, healthcare industry lobbies will work to modify legislation and federal and state regulations to their benefit. However, the direction has been set.

The growth in healthcare expenditures as a percent of GDP is unsustainable. Waste has to be addressed.

Containment of healthcare costs is critical to U.S. global competitiveness and to the sustainability of the quality of life for most Americans. The key is to eliminate inefficiencies and duplicative costs, i.e., waste.

U.S. Health Expenditures and Their Share of GDP 1960-2020
(In Billions of U.S. $)

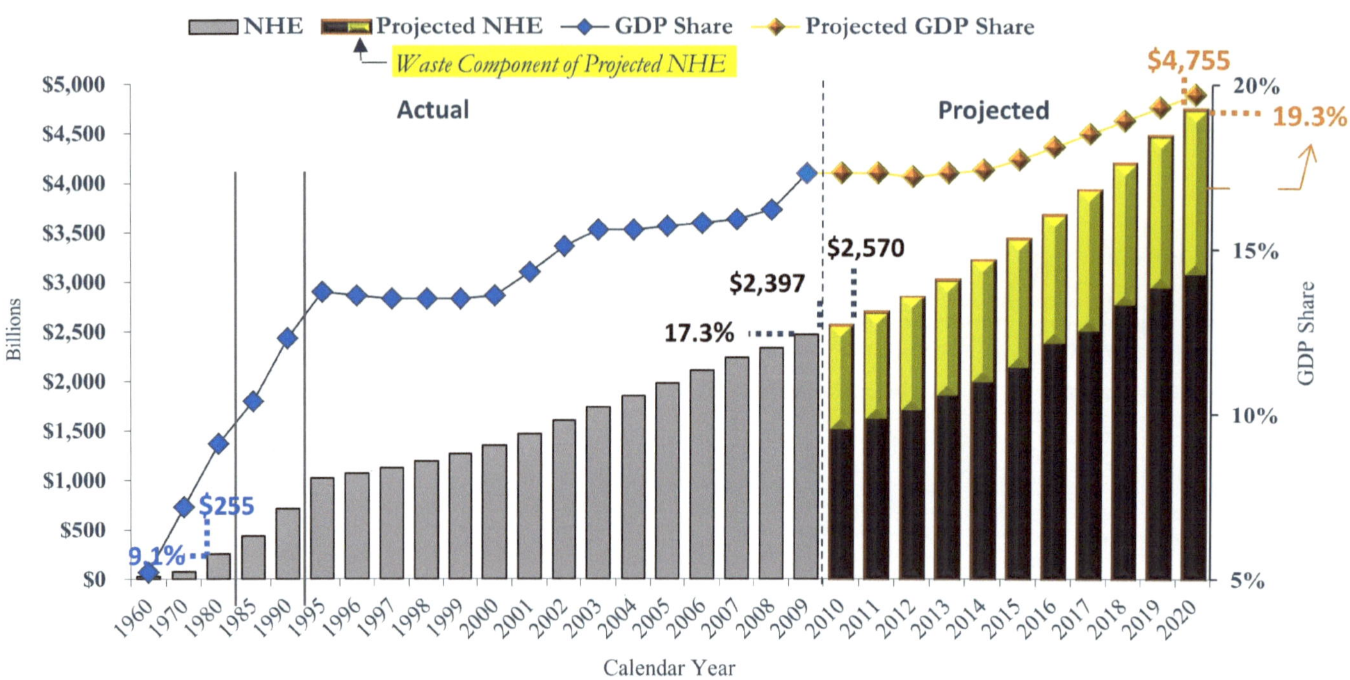

Sources: Centers for Medicare and Medicaid Services, Office of the Actuary, National Health Statistics Group, at http://www.cms.hhs.gov/NationalHealthExpendData/ (Historical data from NHE summary including share of GDP, CY 1960-2008, file nhegdp08.zip; Projected data from NHE Projections 2009-2019, Forecast summary and selected tables, file proj2009.pdf), Wall Street Journal, and 2020 Projection and waste by MMC International.

If something is not done, voters will cast their ballots for new legislators.

From 1990 to 2009, U.S. health insurance premiums increased 3.4 times faster than workers' wages. A new survey from the Center for Studying Health System Change and the Robert Wood Johnson Foundation, released on December 23, 2011, shows the proportion Americans with medical bill-paying difficulty in 2010 was more than one-third higher than in a similar survey in 2003. Overall, the national study shows that one in five Americans reported trouble paying medical bills in 2010. Demand that something be done will only increase.

Cumulative Changes in Health Insurance Premiums, Inflation, and Workers' Earnings, 1999-2009

The growth in healthcare costs and related insurance premiums is unsustainable. They are impacting available disposable income/ quality of life as well as the cost of U.S. products and the ability of the U.S. to compete in world markets.

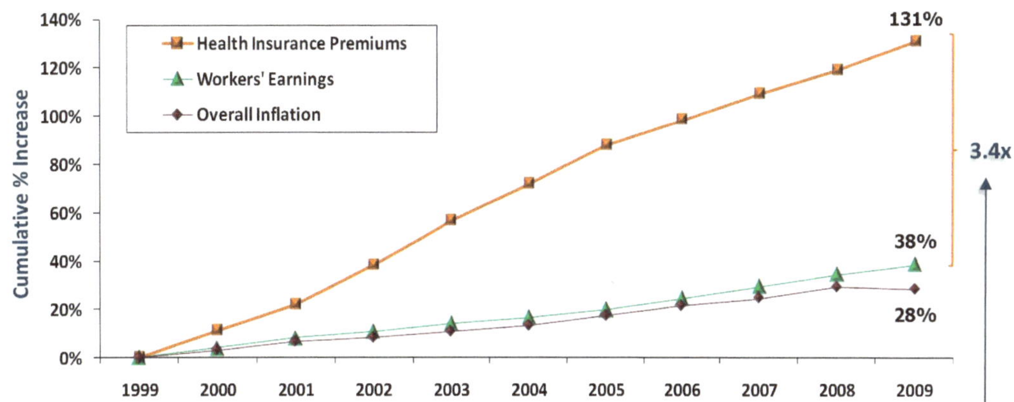

Average Insurance Premiums	1999	2004	2009
Worker's Contribution:	$1,543	$2,661	$3,515
Employer's Contribution:	$4,247	$7,289	$9,860
Total Premium:	**$5,791**	**$9,950**	**$13,375**

Sources: Kaiser/HRET Survey of Employer-Sponsored Health Benefits, 1999-2009. Bureau of Labor Statistics, Consumer Price Index, U.S. City Average of Annual Inflation (April to April), 1999-2009; Bureau of Labor Statistics, Seasonally Adjusted Data from the Current Employment Statistics Survey, 1999-2009 (April to April), and MMC International.

Micromanagement will not work. The focus has to be on enabling competitive market forces.

The unintended consequence of the 1973 HMO Act and passage of DRGs in 1983 was increased costs due to industry fragmentation rather than achieving the healthcare cost-containment objectives the legislation was designed to meet. The only way to extract inefficiencies is to modify or rescind legislation and regulation that impede marketplace completion, offer financial incentives and penalties to encourage providers to decrease costs, and invest in pilot programs to innovate new provider systems and compensation formulas that focus on wellness rather than on procedures.

History Of U.S. Healthcare Legislation

Expansion of health insurance	<1920s	Little known about the treatment of diseases.
	1920s	Doctors and hospitals began charging more than most individuals could easily pay. In turn, hospitals created non-profit health insurance programs– which evolved into Blue Cross.
	1940s	Growth in private insurance accelerated when businesses began offering a health insurance benefit in order to compete for labor and as a way to get around war time wage controls. Government accelerated the trend by exempting healthcare expenses paid by the company from income taxes. To compete for business, private insurers rejiggered premiums by calculating relative risk, and avoided the riskiest potential customers altogether – eliminating the single price system.
	1965	Medicare-Medicaid bill enacted based upon "reasonable and customary" charges. Medicare passed to cover people age ≥65 or who meet other special criteria basically wiped out private insurance for those ≥ 65.
Fragmentation of care	1973	HMO Act of 1973 (began move to managed care)
	1983	Prospective Payment System, DRGs, used by Medicare to pay for hospital care begins move to capitated payments for care.
Towards Universal Coverage	1986	Emergency Medical Treatment and Active Labor Act passed to require hospitals to provide emergency services to everyone, regardless of ability to pay.
	1997	Children's Health Insurance Program (CHIP) cover uninsured children in families with low income that is too high to qualify for Medicaid.
	2003	Medicare Prescription Drug, Improvement, and Modernization Act (MMA) passed to provide a drug benefit as part of Medicare.
	2009	American Recovery and Reimbursement Act's (ARRA) HITECH provisions provide $36B for electronic health records adoption.
	2010	Patient Protection and Affordable Care Act (PPACA) is designed to move the United States as close to universal coverage as possible.

Fragmentation Of U.S. Healthcare

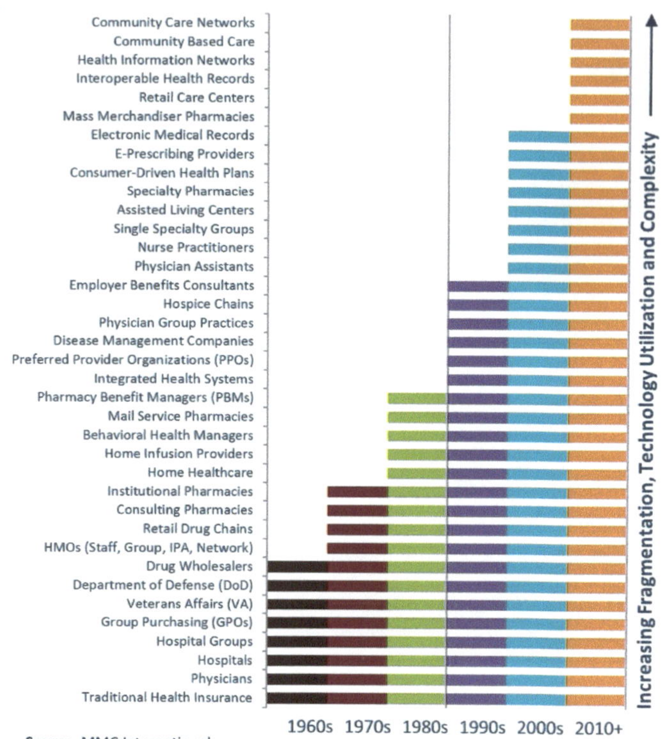

Source: MMC International.

The U.S. is not getting the value it should expect from its healthcare expenditures.

The United States spends >5 percent more of its GDP on healthcare (HC) than any of the other 33 OECD countries - while lagging in a number of quality of care measures, e.g., life expectancy at birth, infant mortality per live births, etc.

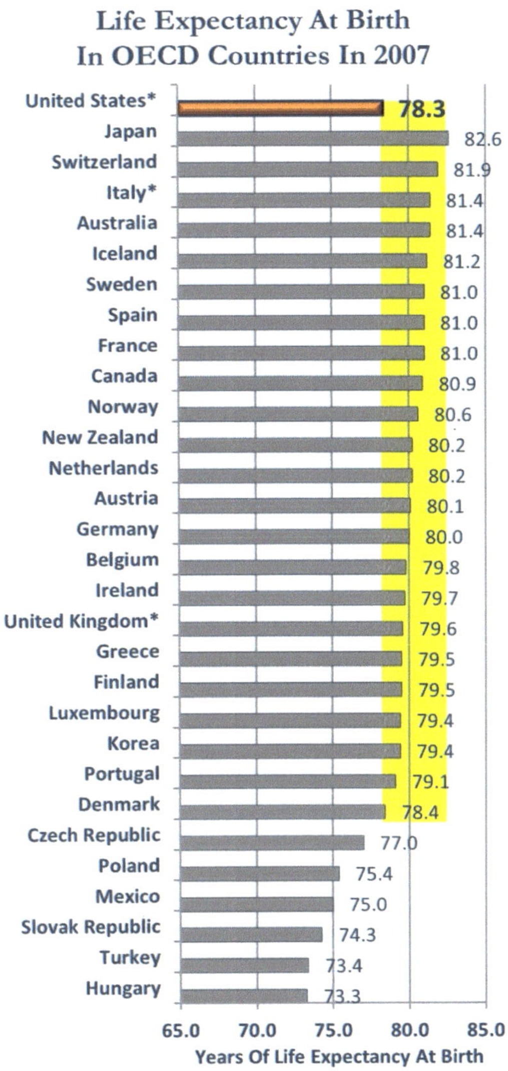

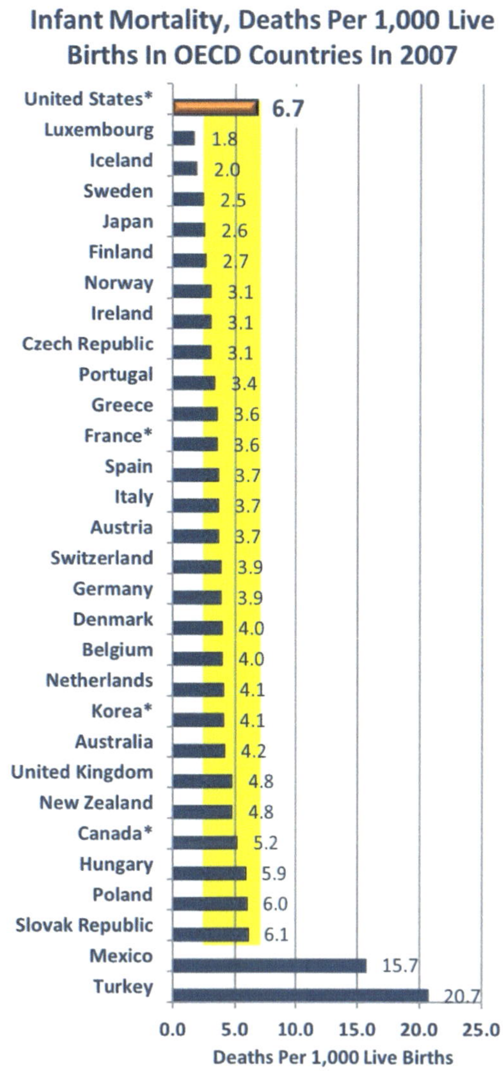

***** = Estimated projection from prior 10 years of data.
OECD = Organization for Economic Cooperation and Development
Sources: OECD Health Data 2009 – Version: November 09 and MMC analysis.

The large uninsured population in part explains America's shorter life spans and greater infant mortality.

A large U.S. uninsured population drives up healthcare costs by foregoing preventative care and delaying care until a condition is more serious and more costly to treat. It contributes to the shorter life spans as serious conditions are diagnosed too late for treatment. According to a Harvard Medical School and Cambridge Health Alliance study, published online in September 2009, American Journal of Public Health, uninsured, working-age Americans have a 40 percent higher risk of death than their privately insured counterparts. Nearly 45,000 annual deaths, one death every 12 minutes, are associated with lack of health insurance, exceeding deaths caused by many common killers such as kidney disease. Lack of health insurance is also felt to contribute to the high U.S. infant mortality rate at birth.

Uninsured U.S. Population
In Millions

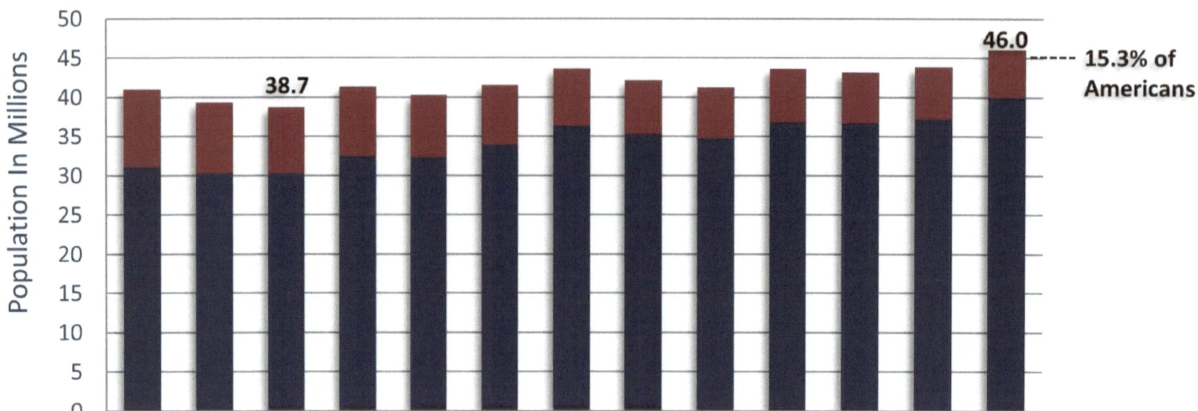

	1997	1998	1999	2000	2001	2002	2003	2004	2005	2006	2007	2008	2009
Under 18	9.9	9.1	8.5	8.9	7.9	7.6	7.3	6.8	6.5	6.8	6.5	6.6	6.1
18 to 64	30.8	30	29.8	32	31.9	33.5	35.9	34.9	34.4	36.5	36.3	37.1	39.7
Over 65	0.3	0.2	0.4	0.4	0.4	0.4	0.4	0.4	0.3	0.3	0.3	0.1	0.2

Data Source: Family Core component of the 1997–2008 NHIS. Data are based on household interviews of a sample of the civilian non-institutionalized population and Martinez, ME and Cohen RA. Health Insurance Coverage: Early Release of Estimates From the National Health Interview Survey, January - September 2009. National Center for Health Statistics, Division of Health Interview Statistics, 2010.

The United States, until enactment of the Patient Protection and Affordable Care Act on March 23, 2010 (PPACA), was the only developed economy and OECD country (with the exception of Mexico and Turkey which are emerging countries) that did not offer universal healthcare coverage to its population.

Higher U.S. healthcare spending is in part caused by unhealthy lifestyles.

Higher U.S. healthcare spending is in part caused by unhealthy lifestyles that lead to chronic conditions. The United States, with its increasingly sedentary lifestyle, is getting heavier. Doubling of obesity between 1987 and 2010 accounts for 20% to 30% of the rise in healthcare spending. The United States is the second most overweight OECD country after Mexico. Obesity leads to high cost to treat and manage chronic conditions.

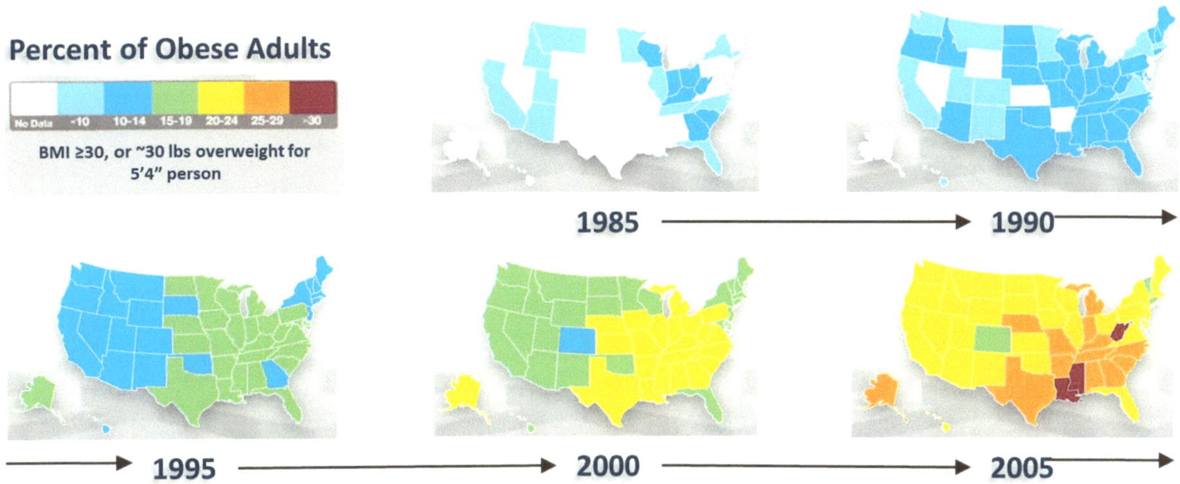

Obesity is not just a problem of appearance. It can worsen, or lead to, a great many other health problems, ranging from minor nuisances like fungal skin infections to life-threatening ones like stroke. Common major diseases that have been linked to obesity include: heart disease, type 2 diabetes, high blood pressure, and cancer.

The following is a list of diseases, organized by body system, that can be caused or worsened by, or are commonly associated with, obesity:

- **Cardiovascular**: Hyperlipidemia, hypercholesterolemia, hypertension, venous stasis disease, atherosclerosis, coronary artery disease, and stroke
- **Endocrine**: Metabolic syndrome, diabetes mellitus type 2
- **Respiratory:** Obstructive sleep apnea, asthma, obesity-hypoventilation syndrome
- **Dermatologic**: fungal skin infections, acanthosis nigricans
- **Nervous**: Migraine, pseudotumor cerebri
- **Gastrointestinal**: Gallbladder disease and gallstones; fatty liver disease (nonalcoholic steatohepatitis or NASH; gastroesophageal reflux disease (GERD), colon cancer, esophageal cancer)
- **Reproductive**: Polycystic ovarian syndrome, breast cancer, endometrial cancer
- **Urologic**: stress incontinence, renal cancer
- **Musculoskeletal**: Osteoarthritis, degenerative joint disease, gout, decreased muscle mass
- **Overweight children** have increased health risks. Type 2 diabetes was once rare in children, but now it accounts for 8% to 45% of newly diagnosed diabetes cases in American children and teens. Overweight children are more likely to remain overweight or become obese as adults.

Sources: Adapted by MMC International from CDC, MedPedia and Partnership to Fight Chronic Disease data and tracking maps.

U.S. Government Programs to change lifestyles have worked. The focus now is on obesity.

The U.S. antismoking campaign has cut the percentage of the U.S. smoking population in half since the mid-1980s. Alcohol consumption in the United States has decreased over 18% since its peak in the early 1980s. The focus, at least through 2020, will be to decrease the U.S. overweight population. Once considered a problem only of high-income countries, obesity rates are rising worldwide. These increases have been felt most dramatically in urban settings. The only remaining region of the world where obesity is not common is sub-Saharan Africa. Obesity is not only a U.S. epidemic.

Percent 15+ Years Old Daily Smokers

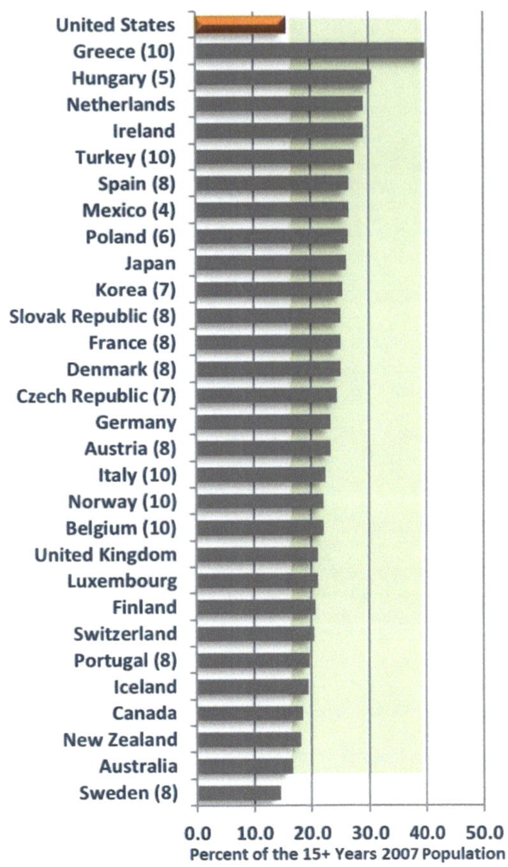

Liters Of Alcohol Per Capita

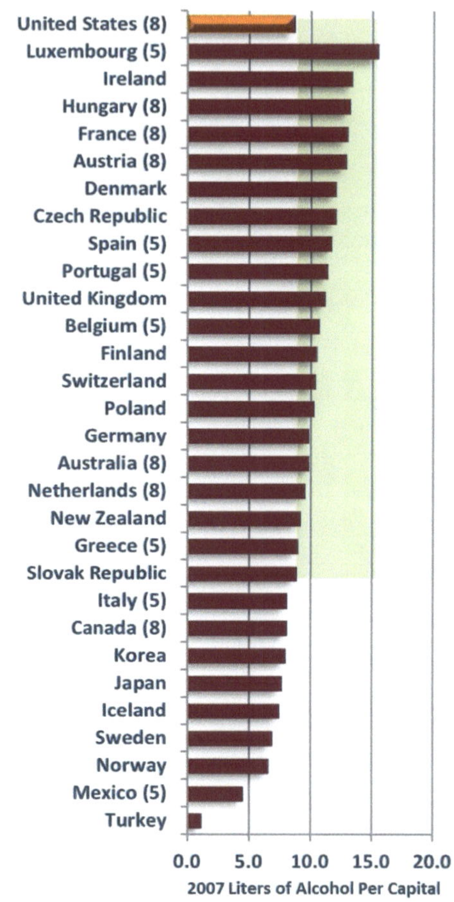

1 = 1999 data; 2 = 2000 data; 3 = 2001 data; 4 = 2002 data; 5 = 2003 data; 6 = 2004 data; 7 = 2005 data; 8 = 2006 data; 10 = 2008 data.
Sources: OECD Health Data 2009 - Version: November 09 and MMC analysis.
Note: Estimates relate to the adult population (normally the population aged 15+) and are based on national health interview surveys for most countries (self-reported data), except for Australia, the Czech Republic (since 2005), Japan, Luxembourg, New Zealand, the Slovak Republic (since 2004), the United Kingdom and the United States where estimates are based on the actual measurement of weight and height. This difference in survey methodologies limits data comparability, as estimates arising from the actual measurement of weight and height are significantly higher than those based on self-report.

The U.S. lags in pediatric preventative healthcare.

Preventive healthcare services improve health by protecting against disease, lessening its impact, or detecting disease at an early stage when it is easier and less expensive to treat – however, the U.S. is lagging in preventive pediatric care behind a number of OECD countries.

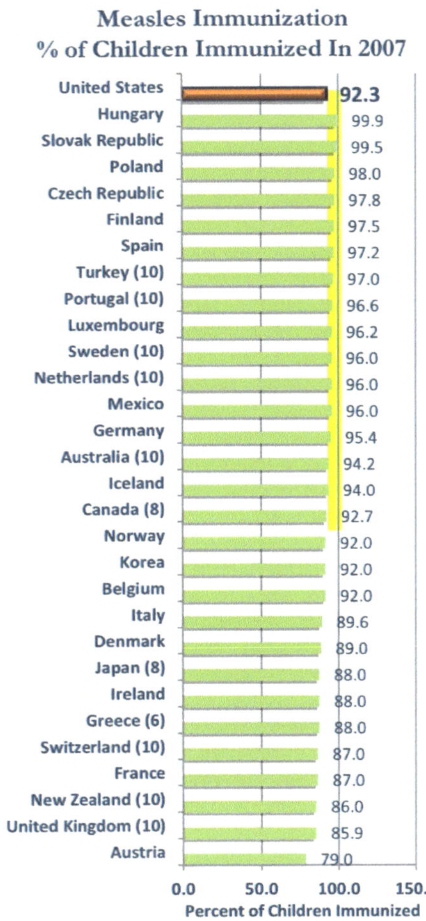

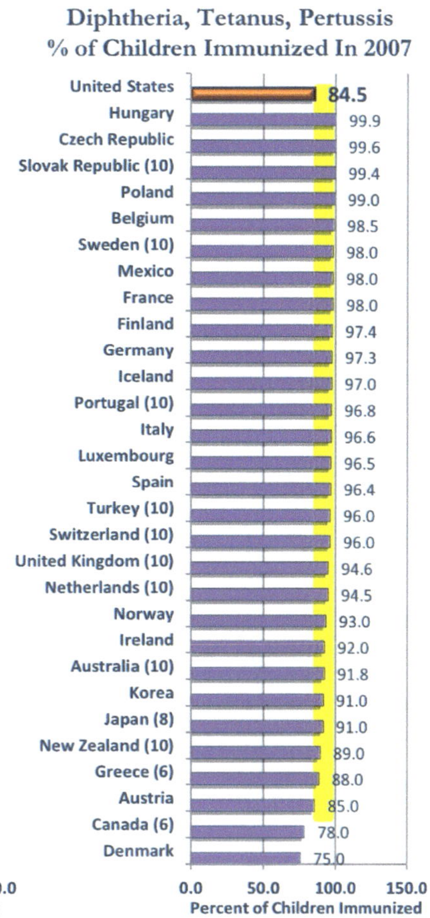

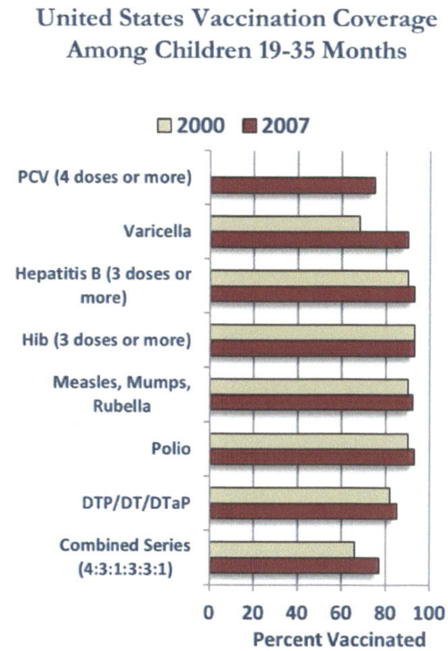

1 = 1999 data; 2 = 2000 data; 3 = 2001 data; 4 = 2002 data; 5 = 2003 data; 6 = 2004 data; 7 = 2005 data; 8 = 2006 data; 10 = 2008 data.
Sources: OECD Health Data 2009 - Version: November 09 and Health, United States, 2009, United States Department of Health and Human Services, Centers for Disease Control and Prevention, National Center for Health Statistics and Health, United States, 2009, U.S. Department of Health and Human Services, Centers for Disease Control and Prevention, National Center for Health Statistics.

In 2007, only 67% of children 19-35 months of age received a combined vaccination series protecting them against seven childhood infectious diseases. Continued effort is required to catch up with the leading developed nations.

The U.S. also lags in preventive care for its adult population…driving up healthcare costs.

Lack of health insurance and lack of coverage for preventative services, such as mammograms, is felt to be responsible for the number of women ≥40 years of age that have not had a mammogram over the last two (2) years.

Influenza Immunizations For ≥65 Years Population In 2007

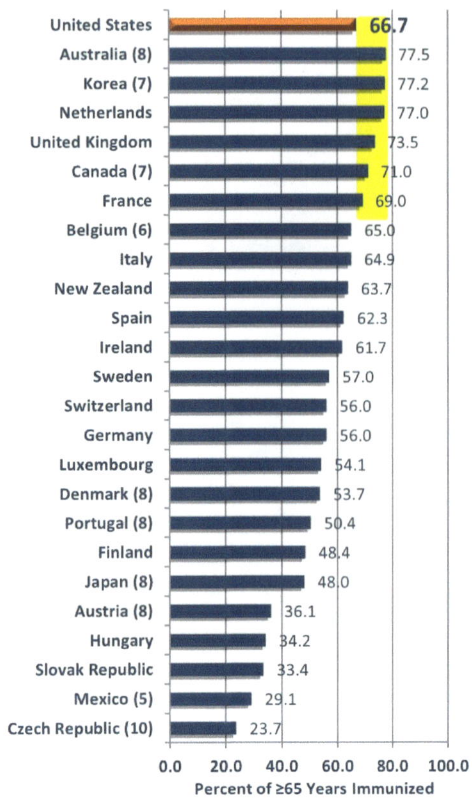
United States 66.7
Australia (8) 77.5
Korea (7) 77.2
Netherlands 77.0
United Kingdom 73.5
Canada (7) 71.0
France 69.0
Belgium (6) 65.0
Italy 64.9
New Zealand 63.7
Spain 62.3
Ireland 61.7
Sweden 57.0
Switzerland 56.0
Germany 56.0
Luxembourg 54.1
Denmark (8) 53.7
Portugal (8) 50.4
Finland 48.4
Japan (8) 48.0
Austria (8) 36.1
Hungary 34.2
Slovak Republic 33.4
Mexico (5) 29.1
Czech Republic (10) 23.7
0.0 20.0 40.0 60.0 80.0 100.0
Percent of ≥65 Years Immunized

United States Women ≥40 Years Of Age Who Had A Mammogram In The Past 2 Years

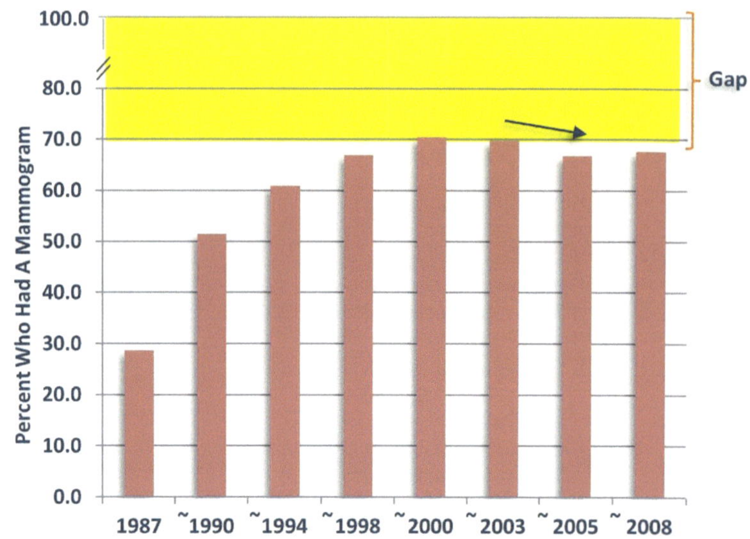

• 5 = 2003 data; 6 = 2004 data; 7 = 2005 data; 8 = 2006 data; 10 = 2008 data.

Sources: OECD Health Data 2009 - Version: November 09 and Health, United States, 2009, United States Department of Health and Human Services, Centers for Disease Control and Prevention, National Center for Health Statistics and Health, United States, 2009, U.S. Department of Health and Human Services, Centers for Disease Control and Prevention, National Center for Health Statistics.

U.S. adoption and higher utilization of costly technologies contribute to higher healthcare costs.

In the United States, between 1996 and 2007, there was more than a three-fold increase in the number of visits per 100 population to physician offices and hospital outpatient departments during which MRI/CT/PET scans were ordered or provided, as well as a four-fold increase in advanced imaging ordered or provided during emergency department visits. Significant increases have also occurred with the utilization of angioplasty utilizing drug-eluting stents, hospitalizations with respiratory intubation and mechanical ventilation, hospital discharges with at least one knee or hip replacement, outpatient cholecystectomies, upper endoscopy (EGD), lower endoscopy (colonoscopy), in-vitro diagnostic testing, kidney and liver transplants, assisted reproductive technology (ART) cycles, and the utilization of drugs to manage heart disease, diabetes, and highly active antiretroviral therapy (HAART) to treat HIV.

CT Scanners Per Million Of Population, 2007*

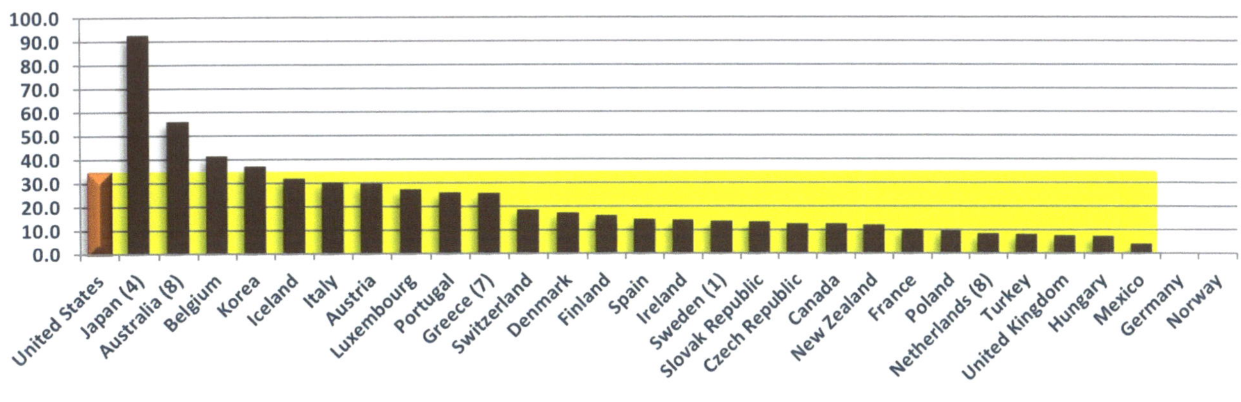

MRI Units Per Million Of Population, 2007*

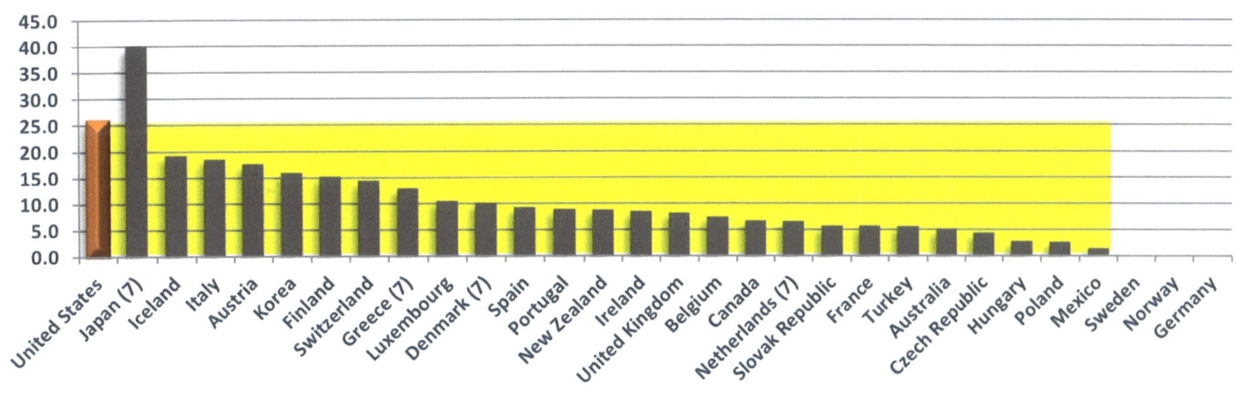

* 1 = 1999 data; 4 = 2002 data; 7 = 2005 data; 8 = 2006 data.

Sources: OECD Health Data 2009 - Version: November 09 and Health, United States, 2009, United States Department of Health and Human Services, Centers for Disease Control and Prevention, National Center for Health Statistics.

Low relative U.S. out-of-pocket expenditures are felt to increase utilization of higher-cost procedures.

Low relative U.S. out-of-pocket expenditures, versus the majority of OECD countries, are felt to lead to increased utilization of higher-cost procedures by the U.S. insured population. Historically, all OECD countries, with the exception of the United States, Mexico and Turkey, provided universal healthcare coverage for their populations. In the United States, the cost for the uninsured is mainly covered by Federal and State governments – with some coming from out-of-pocket payments.

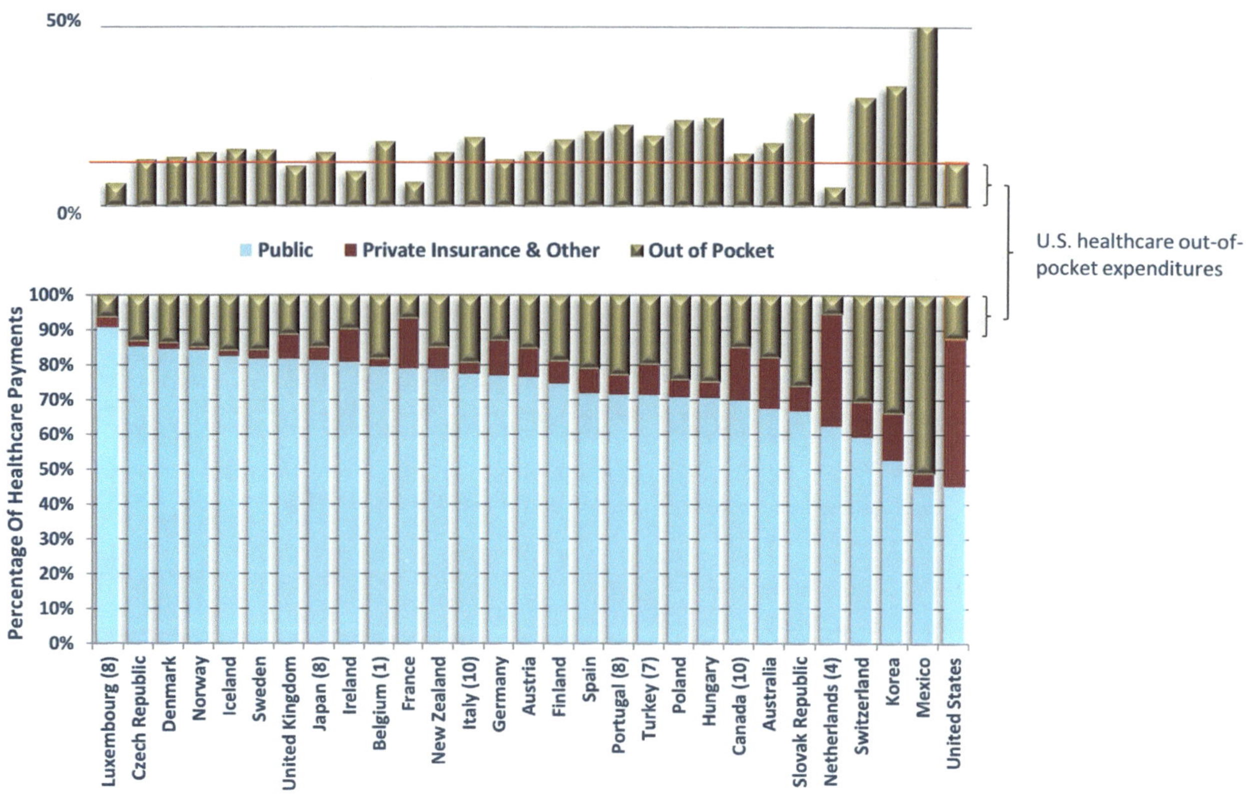

1 = 1999 data; 4 = 2002 data; 7 = 2005 data; 8 = 2006 data; 10 = 2008 data.
Sources: OECD Health Data 2009 - Version: November 09 and MMC analysis.

Health Technology Assessment allows payers to base reimbursement on the best outcomes.

Health Technology Assessments (HTAs) have been utilized in many mature markets for a number of years, but historically not in the United States. The Patient-Centered Outcomes Research Institute (PCORI) was required to be created by September 2010 by the Patient Protection and Affordable Care Act.

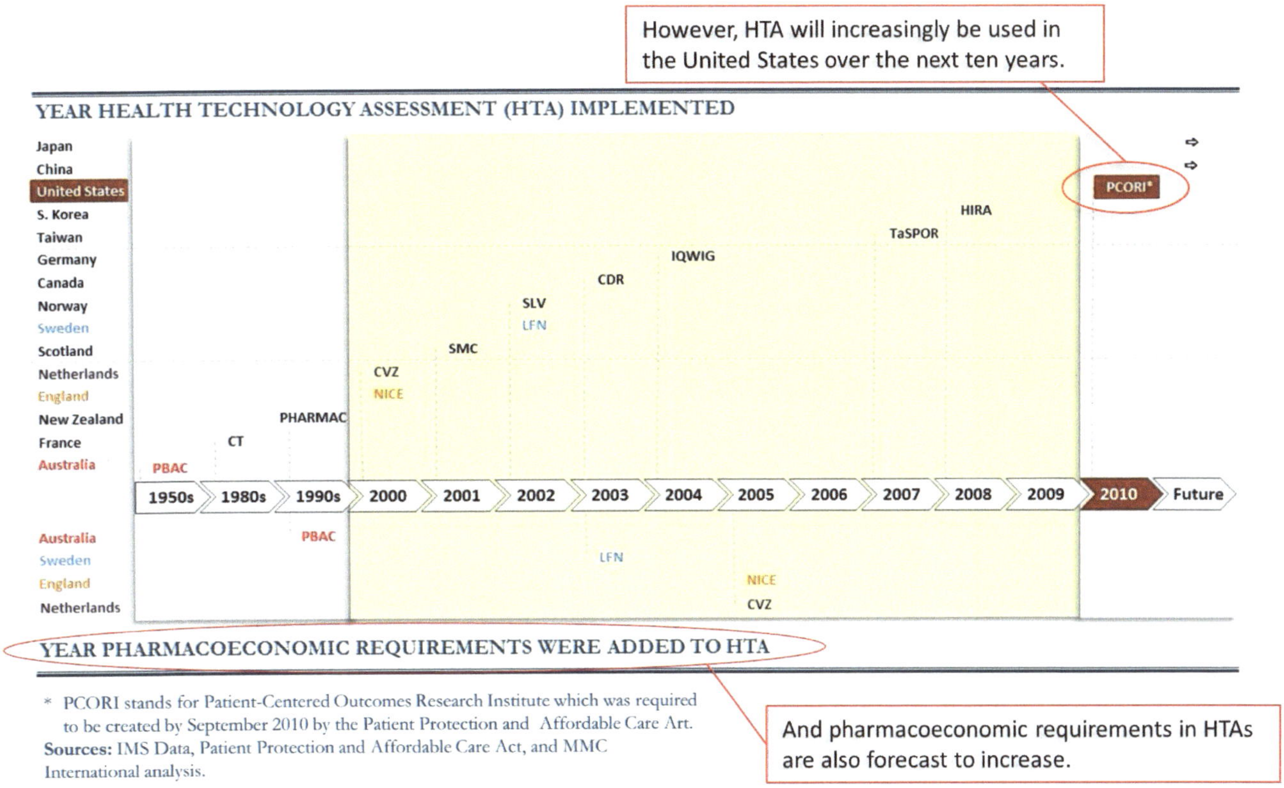

* PCORI stands for Patient-Centered Outcomes Research Institute which was required to be created by September 2010 by the Patient Protection and Affordable Care Art.
Sources: IMS Data, Patient Protection and Affordable Care Act, and MMC International analysis.

Focus will be on management of the patients that consume 75 percent of healthcare expenditures.

Cost containment requires that payers and providers focus on prevention and management of chronic conditions…and efficient management of the critically ill aging population. To contain costs, the focus has to be on managing the 15% of the U.S. population and their chronic diseases that consume >75 percent of healthcare expenditures. Treating heart disease, stroke, cancer, diabetes and mental disorders accounts for about 75 percent of health costs. Trends in chronic conditions management indicate how the U.S. healthcare system will evolve.

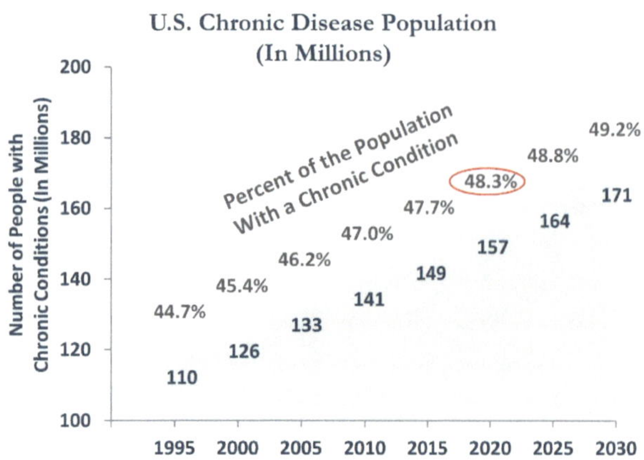

Sources: Ohio Medical Center, CDC, and fightchronicdisease.org

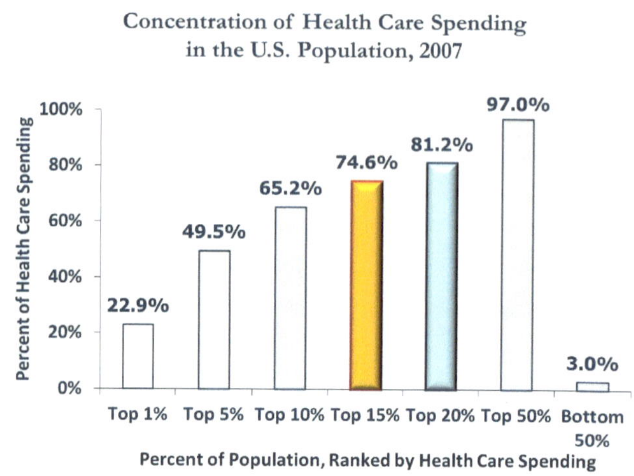

Source: Data from U.S. Department of Health and Human Services, Agency for Healthcare Research and Quality, Medical Expenditure Panel Survey (MEPS), 2007.

- By 2020, nearly half, 48.3%, of the U.S. population will have one or more chronic disease(s).
- Those with chronic diseases account for 81% of hospital admissions; 91% of all prescriptions filled; and 76% of all physician visits.
- The Centers for Disease Control (CDC) estimates that chronic disease management represents 75% of all healthcare spending and is responsible for 70% of deaths.

Chronic diseases such as heart disease, stroke, cancer, diabetes, and arthritis – are among the most common, costly, and preventable of all health problems in the U.S.

- Twenty-five percent of the U.S. community population were reported to have one or more of five major chronic conditions:
  - Mood disorders
  - Diabetes
  - Heart disease
  - Asthma
  - Hypertension
- When the other illnesses are added in, total expenses for people with these five major chronic conditions rise to 49 percent of total healthcare costs.
- Expenses for people with one chronic condition were twice as great as for those without any chronic conditions.
- Spending for those with five or more chronic conditions was about 14 times greater than spending for those without any chronic conditions.

Sources: Druss BG, Marcus SC, Olfson M, et al. Comparing the national economic burden of five chronic conditions. Health Aff (Millwood) 2001; 20(6):233-41; Partnership for Solutions, Johns Hopkins University. Chronic Conditions: Making the Case for Ongoing Care. Prepared for the Robert Wood Johnson Foundation. Baltimore, MD, 2002; Friedman B, Jiang HJ, Elixhauser A, et al. Hospital inpatient costs for adults with multiple chronic conditions. Med Care Res Rev 2006; 63(3):1-20.

The high growth expenditure areas of healthcare are also a logical focus for cost-containment efforts.

Hospital, physician, administrative, and pharmaceuticals cost containment are the logical top priorities for reigning in healthcare costs.

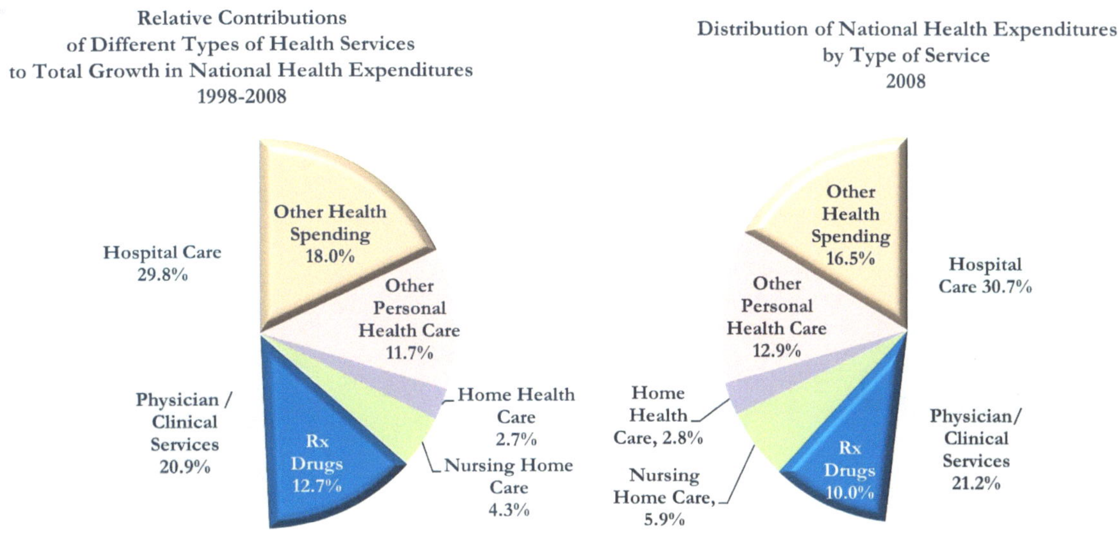

Pharmaceuticals and Other Health Spending (e.g., administration, private health insurance, etc.) were the fastest growing areas of healthcare expenditures between 1998 and 2008.

Note: Other Health Spending includes, for example, administration and net cost of private health insurance, public health activity, research, and structures and equipment, etc. Other Personal Healthcare includes, for example, dental and other professional health services, durable medical equipment, etc.

Sources: NHE data from Centers for Medicare and Medicaid Services, Office of the Actuary, National Health Statistics Group, at http://www.cms.hhs.gov/NationalHealthExpendData/ (see Historical; National Health Expenditures by type of service and source of funds, CY 1960-2008; file nhe2008.zip), and MMC International analysis.

8 UNIVERSAL HEALTHCARE LEGISLATION

Healthcare should be and has historically been a bi-partisan issue.

Compulsory universal healthcare legislation was first proposed during the Democratic presidency of Franklin D. Roosevelt in 1944, by the Social Security Board in its annual report. Republicans introduced a bill in Congress in1949, the Flanders-Ives bill, or the Flanders-Ives-Nixon bill, calling for a federal subsidy to make it possible for low-income people to buy adequate hospital insurance. In 1971, the Nixon Administration proposed a National Health Insurance Standard Act that consisted of two major parts. One part was a government-prescribed minimum amount of private medical and hospital insurance coverage financed by mandatory employer and employee payment of premiums, with a government subsidy of premium payments in specific situations. Healthcare has been and continues as an issue that both the Republican and Democratic parties have to focus upon.

United States universal healthcare coverage has been pursued by both Republicans and Democrats.

United States universal healthcare coverage legislation has a history that goes back to before 1935. It is a non-partisan issue that impacts the life of every American. The Patient Protection and Affordable Care Act (PPACA) incorporates a number of features contained in previous Republican and Democrat championed legislative efforts.

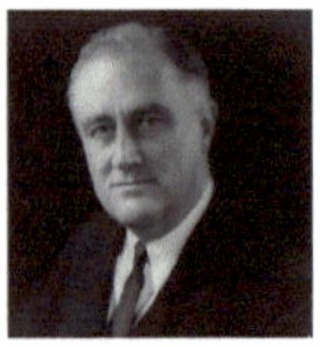

Franklin D. Roosevelt (1933-1945) - Democrat

1935

On Aug. 14, the Social Security Act is signed by Roosevelt. Over the course of the next seven decades, it became one of the most influential, far-reaching health-related acts of Congress in the history of the United States. It eventually served as the legislative launching pad for both Medicare and Medicaid. Shortly after the act became law, FDR appointed the Interdepartmental Committee to Coordinate Health and Welfare Activities to assess the healthcare needs of the American people.

1944

The Social Security Board, in its annual report, recommended compulsory national health insurance.

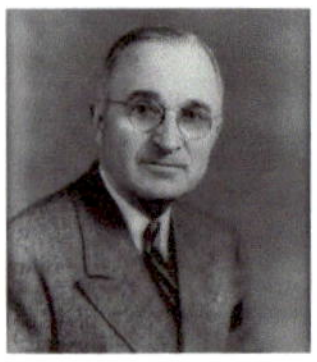

Harry S. Truman (1945-1953) - Democrat

1949

Republicans introduced a bill in Congress, the Flanders-Ives bill, or the Flanders-Ives-Nixon bill, calling for a federal subsidy to make it possible for low-income people to buy adequate hospital insurance. The federal government's proportion of the premium would depend on the individual's income. The states would operate the plan and would be required to share in the cost of the subsidy, depending on the average income in the state. The federal government's share would range from one-third to three-quarters. Hearings were held, but nothing else happened.

1950

The Social Security Act was amended to provide direct payment to doctors, hospitals and other providers of care by the states, with matching federal aid.

1952

Murray-Humphry-Dingell-Celler bills were introduced in the House and Senate calling for health insurance for Social Security beneficiaries.

1952

The President's Commission on Health Needs of the Nation reported in favor of health insurance for Social Security beneficiaries.

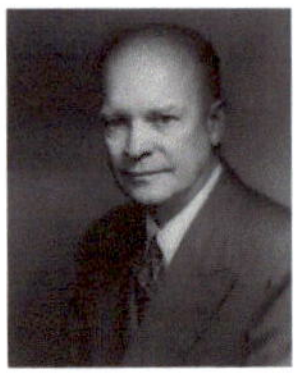

Dwight D. Eisenhower (1953-1961) - Republican

1956

The "Military Medicare" program is enacted, giving healthcare service to military dependents.

1956

The Social Security Act was amended to give monthly benefits to permanently and totally disabled workers between the ages of 50 and 64.

1959

Congress enacted the Federal Employees Health Benefits Act.

1960

The Kerr-Mills bill was passed. It provided federal-state aid for the medically indigent.

1961

The presidential Task Force on Health and Social Security for the American People recommended health insurance for the elderly under Social Security.

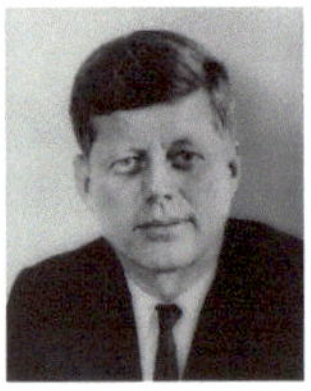

John F. Kennedy (1961-1963) - Democrat

1961

The King-Anderson bill, an early version of Medicare, was introduced in Congress. It did not progress beyond hearings in the Ways and Means Committee.

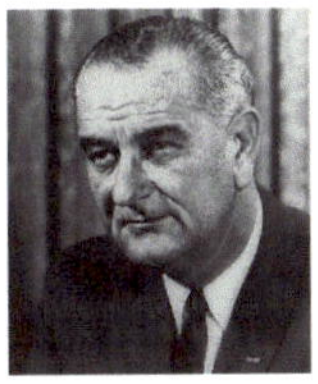

Lyndon B. Johnson (1963-1969) - Democrat

1965

Medicare and Medicaid became part of the Social Security Amendments of 1965 after President Lyndon B. Johnson flew to Independence, Mo., on July 30 to sign the bill into law in the presence of former President Truman, thus ending a stage in the process that had begun several decades before.

1966

Medicare coverage began. All individuals ages 65 and over were automatically covered under Part A. Coverage began for seniors who signed up for the voluntary medical insurance program (Part B). More than 19 million individuals ages 65 and older enrolled in Medicare.

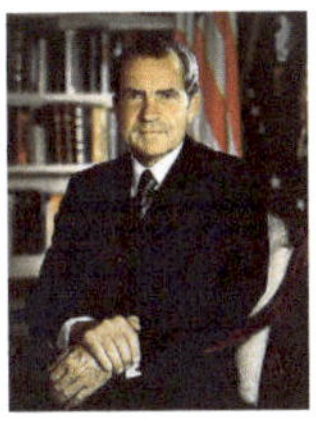

Richard Nixon (1969-1974) - Republican

1971

The Nixon Administration proposed a National Health Insurance Standard Act that consisted of two major parts. One part was a government-prescribed minimum amount of private medical and hospital insurance coverage financed by mandatory employer and employee payment of premiums, with a government subsidy of premium payments in specific situations. The other part was a sliding scale of government-paid benefits for families with earnings less than $5,000 per year.

1972

President Nixon signed the Social Security Amendments of 1972, the first major adjustment to Medicare since its enactment. Medicare eligibility was extended to individuals under age 65 with long-term disabilities (who were receiving SSDI payments for two years) and to individuals with end-stage renal disease.

1973

The HMO Act of 1973 layed the groundwork for managed care. While prepaid group health plans had begun in the early 1900s, this Nixon administration legislation provided federal support to promote their expansion. However, HMOs grew more slowly than anticipated during the 1970s.

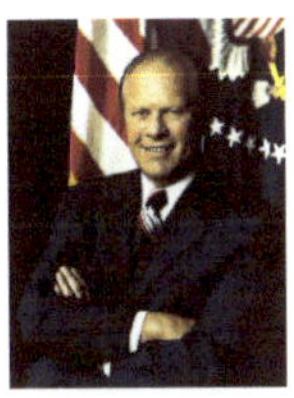

Gerald Ford (1974-1977) - Republican

Other issues superseded the healthcare agenda.

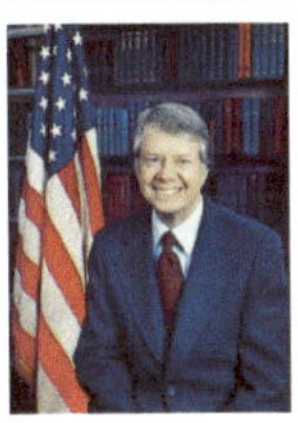

Jimmy Carter (1977-1981) - Democrat

1977

President Carter backed national health insurance when elected to the White House, but other issues soon superseded healthcare.

1980

The Omnibus Reconciliation Act of 1980 expanded home health services by eliminating the limit on the number of home health visits, the prior hospitalization requirement, and the deductible for any Part B benefits. The Baucus Amendments brought Medicare supplemental insurance, also called "Medigap," under federal oversight and established a voluntary certification program for Medigap policies.

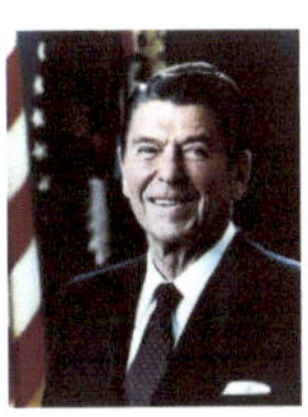

Ronald Reagan (1981-1989) - Republican

1982

The Tax Equity and Fiscal Responsibility Act (TEFRA) increased the Part B premium to cover 25 percent of program costs as part of policies designed to slow the growth of Medicare spending. Hospice services for the terminally ill were added to Medicare's covered benefits. Medicare establishes a risk-based prospective payment system.

1983

In an effort to control Medicare costs and promote efficiency, the inpatient acute hospital prospective payment system was enacted by the federal government. It introduced preset payment rates for treatment of Medicare patients, moving away from reimbursement based on hospital costs. Diagnosis-related groups (DRGs) are developed for payment rate-setting.

1985

The Consolidated Omnibus Budget Reconciliation Act of 1985 made Medicare coverage mandatory for newly hired state and local government employees

1985
The Emergency Medical Treatment and Labor Act is enacted. The law requires any hospital participating in Medicare to provide medical screening and stabilizing treatment to any patient who comes to its emergency room, regardless of ability to pay.
1988
The Medicare Catastrophic Coverage Act of 1988, the largest expansion of the program since the enactment of Medicare, included an outpatient prescription drug benefit and a cap on beneficiaries' out-of-pocket expenses, and expanded hospital and skilled nursing facility benefits. Medicaid began coverage of Medicare premiums and cost-sharing for Medicare beneficiaries with incomes below 100 percent of the federal poverty level, known as Qualified Medicare Beneficiaries. The U.S. Bipartisan Commission on Comprehensive Healthcare (which became known as the Pepper Commission after the late Congressman Claude Pepper of Florida) was established to assess the feasibility of a long-term care benefit under Medicare.

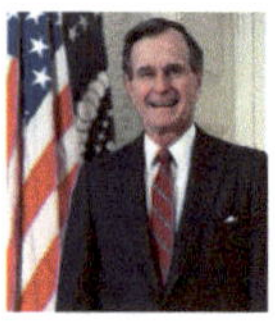

George Bush (1989-1993) - Republican
1989
The Omnibus Budget Reconciliation Act of 1989 establishes the Resource-Based Relative Value Scale for physicians, replacing charge-based payments.
1990
The Omnibus Budget Reconciliation Act of 1990 (OBRA 1990) established the Specified Low-Income Medicare Beneficiary eligibility group requiring state Medicaid programs to cover premiums for beneficiaries with incomes between 100 percent and 120 percent of the federal poverty level. Medicare was expanded to cover screening mammography and partial hospitalization services in community mental health centers. Federal standards were established for Medigap policies, including standardized benefit packages and minimum loss ratios, replacing the voluntary certification system.
1990
The Ryan White Comprehensive AIDS Resources Emergency Act was the single largest federal program designed specifically for people with HIV/AIDS. First enacted in 1990, and reauthorized in 1996 and 2000, the CARE Act provides care and support services to individuals and families affected by HIV/AIDS, functioning as the "payer of last resort"; that is, it fills the gaps in care for those who have no other source of coverage or face coverage limits. Federal CARE Act funding is provided to cities, states and directly to providers and other organizations.

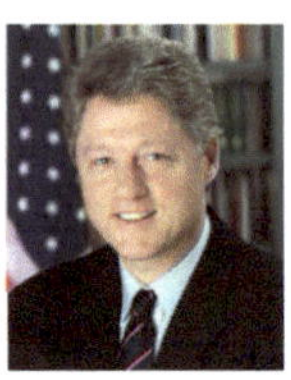

Bill Clinton (1993-2001) - Democrat
1996
The Health Insurance Portability and Accountability Act of 1996 (HIPAA) created national administrative simplification standards for electronic healthcare transactions.
1997
Under the Balanced Budget Act of 1997 (BBA), the State Children's Health Insurance Program (SCHIP) was created.
2000
The Benefits Improvement and Protection Act (BIPA) further increased Medicare payments to providers and managed healthcare organizations, reduced certain Medicare beneficiary co-payments, and improved Medicare's coverage of preventive services.
2000
Authorized by the BBA, the Healthcare Financing Administration implemented an outpatient prospective payment system that significantly changed how hospitals were reimbursed for outpatient services under Medicare.

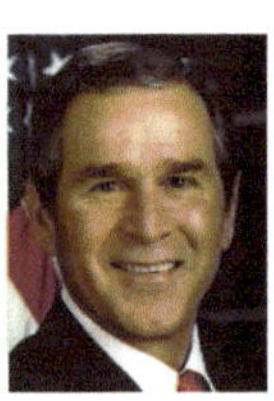

George W. Bush (2001-2009) - Republican
2003
The Medicare Prescription Drug Improvement and Modernization Act (MMA) made the most significant changes to Medicare since the program began. MMA created a prescription drug discount card until 2006, allowed for competition among health plans to foster innovation and flexibility in coverage, covered new preventive benefits and made numerous other changes. In 2006, the new voluntary Part D outpatient prescription drug benefit became available to beneficiaries from private drug plans as well as Medicare Advantage plans. Employers who provide retiree drug coverage comparable to Medicare's became eligible for a federal subsidy.

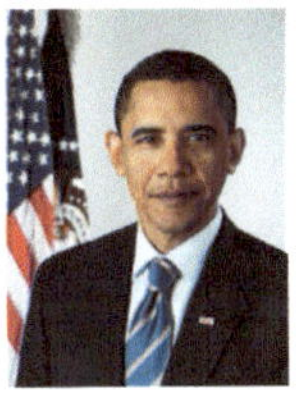

Barack H. Obama (2009-*Present*) – Democrat

2009

The American Reinvestment and Recovery Act (ARRA) made substantial investments to help develop health information technology, expand the primary care workforce and conduct research on comparative effectiveness for healthcare treatment options.

March 23, 2010

The Patient Protection and Affordable Care Act (P.L. 111-148) (also known as PPACA or Affordable Care Act) was enacted. The health reform legislation requires that all individuals have health insurance beginning in 2014.

- The poorest will be covered under a Medicaid expansion.
- Those with low and middle incomes who do not have access to affordable coverage through their jobs will be able to purchase coverage with federal subsidies through new "American Health Benefit Exchanges."
- Employers are not mandated to provide health benefits; however, large businesses whose employees receive insurance subsidies will pay penalties. Small businesses will be able to access more plans through a separate Exchange.
- Health plans will not be allowed to deny coverage to people for any reason, including their health status, nor can they charge more because of a person's health or gender. Young adults will now have the option of being covered under their parents' plan up to age 26.

9 PATIENT PROTECTION AND AFFORDABLE CARE ACT (PPACA)

U.S. healthcare in 2020 will be radically different than it is today.

PPACA legislation was signed into law on March 23, 2010, mandated implementing regulation will continue through 2016, and "execution" through 2020 – unleashing an unprecedented period of innovation, discontinuities and opportunities through at least 2020. The only certainty is that payers, providers and suppliers will innovate to retain or grow their respective revenues/market shares, industry norms will change, a few strategically-driven healthcare companies/entities in each healthcare industry sector will prosper, and wealth will be created. Those that fail to adapt will suffer from decreasing performance which will lead to decreased valuations which will make them vulnerable and limit their strategic options to invest to reposition themselves. Many healthcare companies will be acquired, merged or driven out of business. U.S. healthcare in 2020 will be radically different than it is today. A key driver has been the passage of PPACA.

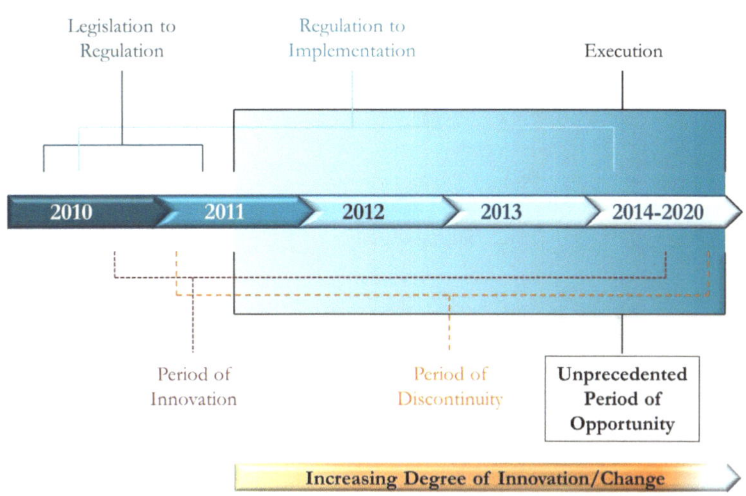

Source: MMC International

PPACA is designed to be implemented by 2018 in 92 coordinated steps.

PPACA implementation was designed to be accomplished via 92 implementation steps that will touch every participant in the U.S. Healthcare System. PPACA is designed to use regulation, incentives and penalties to fundamentally change the way healthcare is viewed, purchased, reimbursed, delivered and managed in the United States. The impact will be stakeholder specific. Industry participants have been and are busy preparing for or reacting to changes in regulation, mandates, and incentives. While politicians argue about repeal and implementation, beneath the political battle lies a success story of early implementation. Since passage of PPACA, the federal and many state governments have been turning major elements of the legislation into reality right on schedule.

Legend

- Affordability and Subsidies
- Employers
- Financing and Taxes
- Fraud and Abuse
- Insurance
- Long-Term Care
- Medicaid and CHIP
- Medical Malpractice
- Medicare
- Prescription Drugs
- Prevention
- Quality
- Workforce

2010 (25 Steps)

- Review of Health Plan Premium Increases
- Changes in Medicare Provider Rates
- Medicaid and CHIP Payment Advisory Commission
- Comparative Effectiveness Research
- Prevention and Public Health Fund
- Medicare Beneficiary Drug Rebate
- Small Business Tax Credits
- Medicaid Drug Rebate
- Coordinating Care for Dual Eligibles
- Generic Biologic Drugs
- New Requirements on Non-profit Hospitals
- Medicaid Coverage for Childless Adults
- Reinsurance Program for Retiree Coverage
- Pre-existing Condition Insurance Plan
- New Prevention Council
- Consumer Website
- Tax on Indoor Tanning Services
- Expansion of Drug Discount Program
- Adult Dependent Coverage to Age 26
- Consumer Protections in Insurance
- Insurance Plan Appeals Process
- Coverage of Preventive Benefits
- Health Centers and the National Health Service Corps
- Health Care Workforce Commission
- Medicaid Community-Based Services

2011 (21 Steps)

- Minimum Medical Loss Ratio for Insurers
- Closing the Medicare Drug Coverage Gap
- Medicare Payments for Primary Care
- Medicare Prevention Benefits
- Center for Medicare and Medicaid Innovation
- Medicare Premiums for Higher-Income Beneficiaries
- Medicare Advantage Payment Changes
- Medicaid Health Homes
- Chronic Disease Prevention in Medicaid
- CLASS Program
- National Quality Strategy
- Changes to Tax-Free Savings Accounts
- Grants to Establish Wellness Programs
- Teaching Health Centers
- Medical Malpractice Grants
- Funding for Health Insurance Exchanges
- Nutritional Labeling
- Medicaid Payments for Hospital-Acquired Infections
- Graduate Medical Education
- Medicare Independent Payment Advisory Board
- Medicaid Long-Term Care Services

2012 (10 Steps)

- Accountable Care Organizations in Medicare
- Medicare Advantage Plan Payments
- Medicare Independence at Home Demonstration
- Medicare Provider Payment Changes
- Fraud and Abuse Prevention
- Annual Fees on the Pharmaceutical Industry
- Medicaid Payment Demonstration Projects
- Data Collection to Reduce Health Care Disparities
- Medicare Value-Based Purchasing
- Reduced Medicare Payments for Hospital Readmissions

2013 (13 Steps)

- State Notification Regarding Exchanges
- Closing the Medicare Drug Coverage Gap
- Medicare Bundled Payment Pilot Program
- Medicaid Coverage of Preventive Services
- Medicaid Payments for Primary Care
- Itemized Deductions for Medical Expenses
- Flexible Spending Account Limits
- Medicare Tax Increase
- Employer Retiree Coverage Subsidy
- Tax on Medical Devices
- Financial Disclosure
- CO-OP Health Insurance Plans
- Extension of CHIP

Legend

- Affordability and Subsidies
- Employers
- Financing and Taxes
- Fraud and Abuse
- Insurance
- Long-Term Care
- Medicaid and CHIP
- Medical Malpractice
- Medicare
- Prescription Drugs
- Prevention
- Quality
- Workforce

2014 (20 Steps)

- Expanded Medicaid Coverage
- Presumptive Eligibility for Medicaid
- Individual Requirement to Have Insurance
- Free Choice Vouchers
- Health Insurance Exchanges
- Health Insurance Premium and Cost Sharing Subsidies
- Guaranteed Availability of Insurance
- No Annual Limits on Coverage
- Essential Health Benefits
- Multi-State Health Plans
- Temporary Reinsurance Program for Health Plans
- Basic Health Plan
- Employer Requirements
- Medicare Advantage Plan Loss Ratios
- Wellness Programs in Insurance
- Fees on Health Insurance Sector
- Medicare Independent Payment Advisory Board Report
- Medicare Disproportionate Share Hospital Payments
- Medicaid Disproportionate Share Hospital Payments
- Medicare Payments for Hospital-Acquired Infections

2015 (One Step)

- Increase Federal Match for CHIP

2016 (One Step)

- Health Care Choice Compacts

2018 (One Step)

- Tax on High-Cost Insurance

Sources: Adapted By MMC International from Henry J. Kaiser Foundation information/graphics.

The focus is on:

- Universal coverage – to reduce premature deaths and costly preventable conditions
- Lifestyle changes – because 70% of healthcare costs are preventable
- Focus on prevention – chronic diseases can be prevented or managed
- Accountable Care Organizations – reduce provider inefficiencies
- Reimbursement changes – to focus on wellness rather than procedures
- Health Insurance – to increase competition to reduce costs
- Electronic Health Records – decrease duplicative care, disseminate best practices and improve outcomes
- Benchmarking – allow comparative shopping and outcomes reimbursement
- Comparative Studies – reimburse for what works/for value – evidence-based medicine
- Increase the number of nurses, primary care physicians and certain specialists.

The objective is to increase the quality of care and the wellness of the population while simultaneously decreasing costs.

10 CONSUMERS

Consumer demands will affect all aspects of U.S. healthcare.

Between 2012 and 2020, consumers, which are wealthier, more educated and more connected than their parents, will become increasingly more involved in their healthcare. They will fundamentally transform how and where patients are diagnosed, screened, treated, and diseases monitored and managed. They will also shift where and how care is delivered. They will influence product and therapy choices for many products. They will shape the political agenda.

Family healthcare premiums have risen faster than the Consumer Price Index (CPI).

Since 2004, family healthcare premiums have risen over 2.5 times faster than the Consumer Price Index (CPI). As a result, employers have been increasing worker premium contributions - negatively impacting disposable income and many Americans' quality of life. According to *The Harris Poll* by Harris Interactive, in 2010, 45 percent of the American population believed healthcare was the most important issue for the government to address. The increasing consumer healthcare burden will result in increasing pressure for the government and payers to contain healthcare costs.

Most Important Issues For Government To Address

Spontaneous, unprompted replies

By Percent of U.S. Adult Population

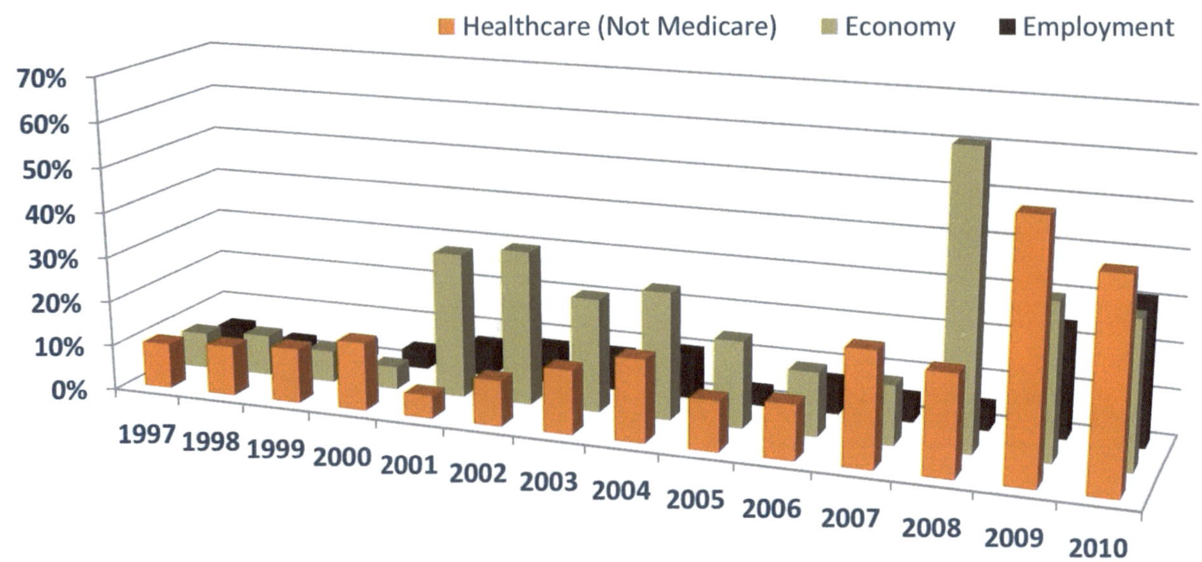

Sources: Adapted by MMC International from *The Harris Poll* by Harris Interactive, May 1997, Jan 1998, Feb 1999, Aug 2000, Dec 2001, Dec 2002, Jun 2003, Oct 2004, Aug 2005, Jun 2006, Oct 2007, Oct 2008, Nov 2009, Jan 2010.

Cumulative Change in Family Premiums and CPI 1999-2009

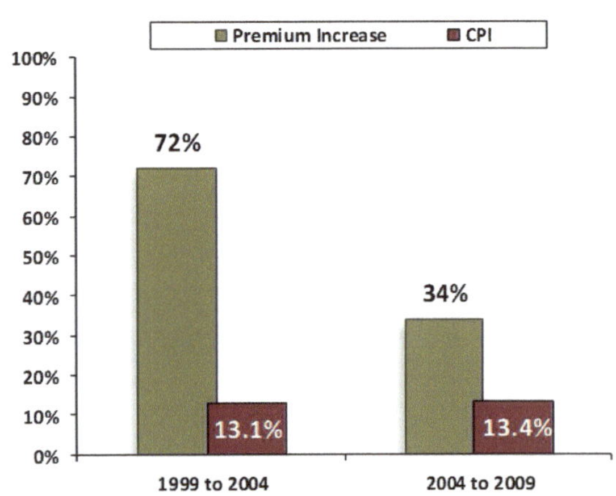

Source: Kaiser/HRET Survey of Employer-Sponsored Health Benefits, 1999-2009. Bureau of Labor Statistics, Consumer Price Index, U.S. City Average of Annual Inflation (April to April), 1999-2009.

- Healthcare costs are decreasing individual and family disposable income. They are negatively impacting American's quality of life.
- By 2014, under PPACA legislation, individuals are required to have qualifying health insurance or face a tax penalty.
  - This means an incremental 32 million will join the insurance roles and will join the ranks of those concerned about rising healthcare costs.
  - This provision is at the heart of Republican challenges to PPACA.
    - Regardless of the outcome to legal challenges regarding the requirement of individuals to purchase health insurance or pay a penalty, pressures will continue to reduce healthcare costs.

PPACA's major provisions appear to be very popular with the public.

With a few notable exceptions -- such as requiring that people have insurance – PPACA's major provisions appear to be very popular with the public. If history repeats itself, if healthcare reform continues on pace, as happened with Part D, the law's fate will be determined not by the early political debate but by how people believe the law is working for them and their families and friends once its major elements are implemented.

The government has made substantial progress beginning six months after PPACA passage in implementing reform, including many measures popular with the public...

- No pre-existing condition exclusions for children (72% favorable)
- Extend dependent coverage to age 26 (53% favorable)
- No out-of-pocket costs for preventative services (70% favorable)
- No cancellation of coverage except for fraud (68% favorable)
- High risk pool for people with pre-existing conditions (61% favorable)
- Small business health insurance tax credits (71% favorable)
- Drug rebates for Medicare beneficiaries (64% favorable)

...but major elements of the law that will affect many more people don't kick in until 2014.

- Guaranteed access to insurance regardless of your health (69% favorable)
- Insurance exchanges to make it easier to buy coverage (87% favorable)
- Tax credits to make insurance more affordable for low and middle income people (76% favorable)
- Expanded Medicaid coverage for low income people (71% favorable)
- A requirement that people have insurance (70% UNFAVORABLE)
- Penalties for employers that do not offer coverage to workers (51% favorable, 47% unfavorable)

Consider what happened when a Republican-controlled Congress created the Medicare drug benefit in 2004. Three times as many seniors opposed the law as favored it, and many liberals criticized the legislation as a first step toward privatization of Medicare, just as some conservatives call current health reform a government takeover. Within three years, though, supporters of Medicare Part D outnumbered detractors as it became clear the program was working well and helping seniors afford their medicines. The new health-reform law represents a much bigger change than the Medicare drug benefit was and may work out differently, especially if Republicans succeed in their efforts to block full implementation. But if the reform continues on pace, as happened with Part D, the law's fate will be determined not by the early political debate but by how people believe the law is working for them and their families and friends once its major elements are implemented.

While the politics of health reform remain as ugly as ever, implementation of the law's benefits and changes has been a success story so far. In turn, it has set the direction of healthcare system change.

11 PAYERS

What Medicare does, the rest of the industry will follow.

Growth in total U.S. healthcare expenditures is forecast to grow 79 percent, from $2.6 trillion in 2010 to $4.6 trillion in 2020. During the same time, Federal and State healthcare programs will increase from representing 56 percent, $1.5 trillion, in 2010 to $2.8 trillion, 60 percent of U.S. healthcare expenditures in 2020. The federal and state governments have the concentrated purchasing power, versus Private Insurance and Consumers, to influence both the direction and speed of healthcare change in the United States. PPACA serves as a roadmap relative to the issues and priorities the healthcare industry can expect to encounter between 2012 and 2020.

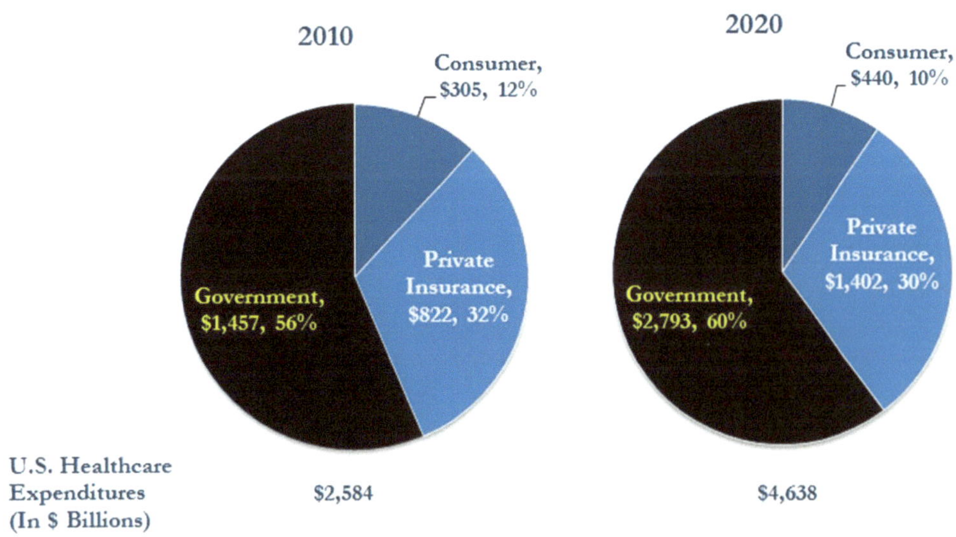

1 2010 Health spending projections and 2020 Forecast were based on the National Health Expenditures (NHE) released in January 2011. The 2020 forecast include impacts from the PPACA (Affordable Care Act).

2 Private Insurance includes Private Health Insurance (Employer Sponsored Insurance, State Health Insurance Exchanges, and other private insurance), Medicare, Medicaid, Children's Health Insurance Program (Titles XIX and XXI), Department of Defense, and Department of Veterans' Affairs.

3 Government includes Children's Health Insurance Program (Titles XIX and XXI), Department of Defense, and Department of Veterans' Affairs, worksite healthcare, other private revenues, Indian Health Service, workers' compensation, general assistance, maternal and child health, vocational rehabilitation, other federal programs, Substance Abuse and Mental Health Services Administration, other state and local programs, and school health.

Source: Compiled by MMC International from data provided by the Centers for Medicare & Medicaid Services, Office of the Actuary.

12 COST EXTRACTIONS

The focus on extracting costs/inefficiencies will fundamentally shift market forces in many sectors.

Any entity or service that stands between the healthcare provider and the patient must be able to justify their existence by cost effectively adding value to the system – either a lower cost or a better outcome or both. The following graphic depicts key healthcare sectors that stand between healthcare providers and the patient. Legislation and regulation need to be changed to enable market competition to drive out system inefficiencies and high costs. Duplication in administration, systems, processes, equipment, facilities, insurance, high prices, etc. need to be extracted. Product purchases based upon medical and/or cost effectiveness will drive new technologies, innovations, and cost extractions from suppliers. Intermediaries, such as wholesalers and buying groups, will have to cost justify their offerings.

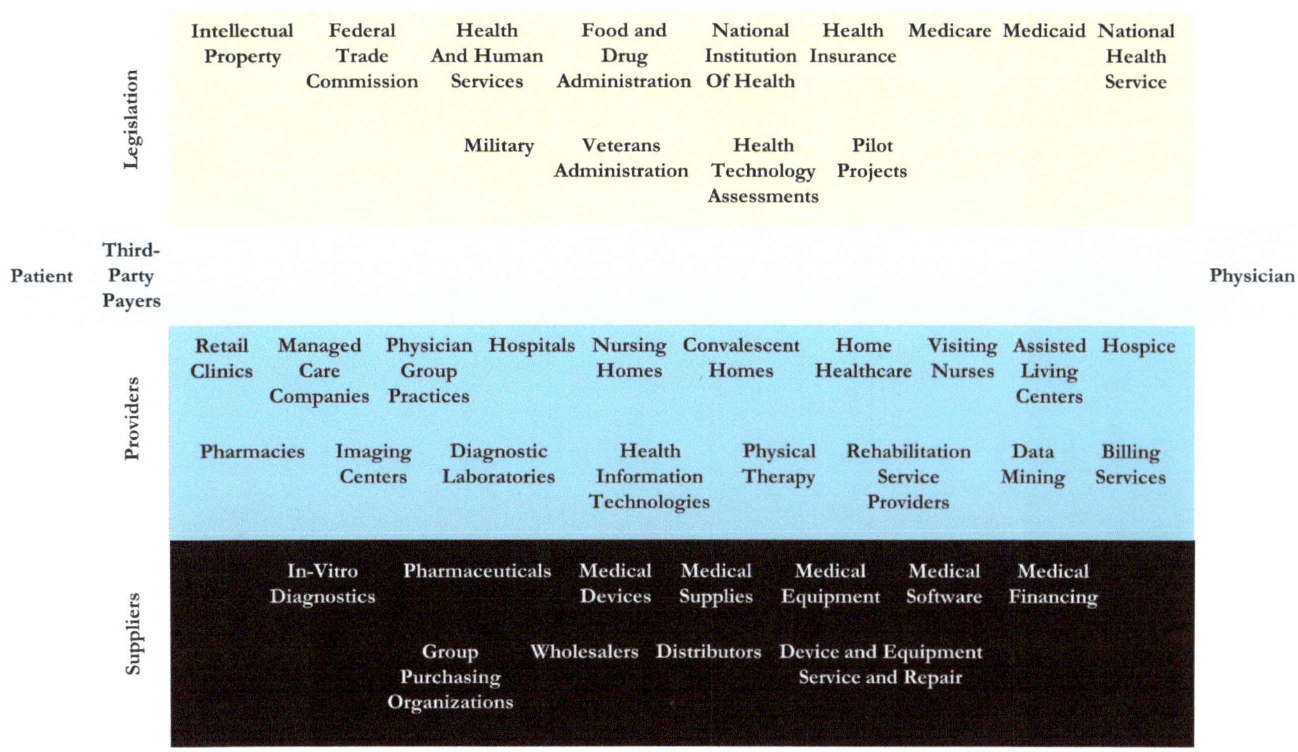

A critical key to unleashing costs from the U.S. healthcare system will be to remove artificial barriers that provide protection from competition and preclude marketplace forces from extracting inefficiencies without returns to consumers, payers, and/or taxpayers. Regardless of the speed of legislative and regulatory change, payers and providers will be looking at ways to extract costs to capture or maintain competitive advantage – causing participants to innovate to maintain or increase share – thereby driving industry discontinuities and opportunities.

13 MARKET AND INDUSTRY LIFECYCLES

A number of factors indicate where an industry and/or market is in its lifecycle.

All markets and industries go through lifecycles. Lifecycles are driven by innovation, new products, competition, customers, financial requirements and cash flows. Each market has its own competitive boundaries, e.g., local, regional, national or global. All industries, markets and products eventually mature and persist until a new technology, innovation and/or product is introduced to redefine the traditional industry, market and/or product, i.e., film processing by digital pictures, ocean liners by airplanes, personal workstations by portable computers, music records by digitalized music, etc. Each phase of the lifecycle carries its own risk and rewards, evidences its own traits, has different investment requirements, and demands its own strategies.

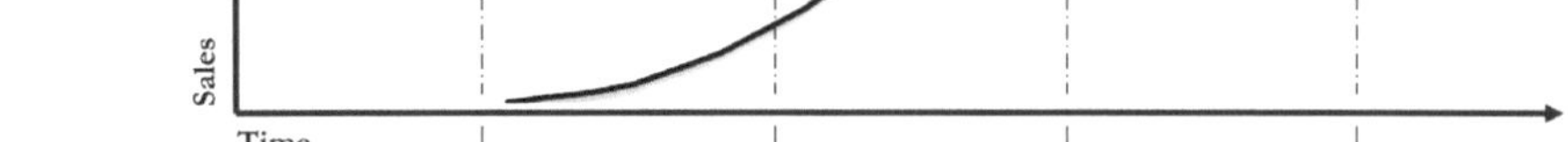

	Development	Emerging	Growth	Maturity	Decline
Risk	Medium	High / Medium	Medium / Low	Low / High	Low
Strategy	Develop Product Portfolio	Secure Market Position	Capture Dominant Market Position	Redeploy Resources (Higher Return Areas)	Focus on Free Cash Flows
Resource Allocation	Invest	Invest	Invest	Maintain/Harvest	Harvest

In a mature market, you have to be number one or number two to make a profit.

An empirical observation indicates that in a stable competitive market when the number one company in any market has twice the share of the number two company and four times the share of the rest of the competitors combined that it does not behoove any competitor to try to increase share. At this point, the cost differential produces very large profits for the market leader at breakeven prices for the low share competitor. The differential is enough to discourage further reinvestment and efforts to compete by the low share competitors unless the leader is willing to lose share by holding a price umbrella. At this juncture, competition has decreased pricing to the point where the market leader's profitability equals its risk adjusted return on capital. For the market leader, this means that at this equilibrium other investments with higher growth prospects will yield higher returns than investments to increase market share. This is counterintuitive as this is the point where the top two companies are throwing off the most cash flow. Any competitor with less than one quarter the market share of the largest competitor cannot be an effective competitor. "The underlying logic is straightforward. Cost is a function of market share as a result of the experience curve effect" – costs go down as volumes multiply. The cash cycle is an investment cycle. Net cash goes in from the beginning. The net cash input requirement increases with success until the market begins to mature. At that point, cash flows from operations exceed reinvestment requirements. However, the return flow of cash never starts for those who fail to become leaders in their market sector. Absent of outside intervention, e.g., legislation or regulation, they lose their investment.

.

Competition follows the money.

The introduction of a new product requires significant investments in product development, scale-up, market development and market launch. By necessity, this requires a high price, which initially does not cover costs. As the market takes off, costs begin to go down faster than managements are generally willing to decrease price. This creates a price umbrella. At a certain point, the financial community takes note that competing products or companies can be formed which can charge a lower price while making very attractive margins. In turn, financial support allows competitors to begin entering the market. This has the effect of both growing the market and driving prices and costs downward. At a certain point, competitor failures begin to materialize, spooking the financial community and drying up financing. At this same time, many companies with successful offerings need more capital to sustain growth. This is also the point where: 1) there are a number of companies with products or technologies but little cash, 2) a number of companies with cash but no products or technologies (due to failures), and 3) a very few companies with both product and/or technologies plus sufficient financing. Financial necessity results in the beginning of a consolidation phase during the market growth cycle. The outcome of the shakeout is fewer but stronger competitors. Investments continue until growth begins to slow. At this point, new products and/or technologies are not able to offset the decreasing revenues as a result of product portfolio commoditization. Companies that begin experiencing decreasing growth and profitability suffer lower valuations versus stronger competitors. The valuation differential positions industry/market leaders to acquire competitors at a discount – making the acquisitions attractive. Absent of government intervention, consolidation of the maturing market continues until the market is dominated by two companies, the first that has twice the share of the second and four times the share of the rest. At this point the market is mature.

As a market matures, power shifts from the originators/manufacturers to customers.

When a product is exclusive or the market is characterized by a very limited number of competitors, pricing power resides with the innovator/manufacturer. Negotiating power begins to equalize when product substitutes become available - allowing customers choice based upon product features and benefits. Power shifts to customers when products become generic/commodities. Generic product placement and purchasing, everything being equal, is based upon price. Only low-cost competitors are able to profitably compete in commodity markets. This situation continues until a new product offering is introduced that obsolesces the current commodity/generic.

Effective managements obsolesce their products before competitors do.

All technologies and products have their limits. At a certain point incremental investments will not generate new products or incremental product improvements. Technology and product investments get above competitive returns until they hit their productivity limitation. This occurs somewhere around midpoint of the technology or product lifecycle. To maximize shareholder returns, managements have to shift investments in existing technologies and/or products to new technologies and replacement products when these investments begin to evidence decreasing returns. This is counterintuitive because these are the technologies and/or products that are producing the greatest returns. However, managements' key responsibility is to balance the investment portfolio to insure that the company obsolesces its own technologies and/or products before competitors do. This insures a stream of new product offerings designed to insure the continuity/sustainability of the business/enterprise. Companies that fail to properly manage their portfolio investments eventually suffer suboptimal valuations and are either acquired, merged or driven out of business.

As industries mature, the need for intermediaries significantly decreases.

In any industry, intermediary companies materialize when they see an opportunity to provide a service which a company cannot cost competitively do it themselves. These are services which industry participants require. As long as there are multiple competitors and the market/industry is not mature, no individual company has the requisite volume to justify independently investing in the service since intermediaries can spread costs over multiple customers. The intermediary companies generally use the initial platform to begin offering and bundling more services into their pricing. This is their growth phase. This persists until customer industry segments begin to consolidate and individual companies begin to get large enough to drive prices down and to begin to demand unbundling of the services provided by the intermediary. While intermediaries resist unbundling their services, the customers represent a significantly large enough portion of their business that they comply with the unbundling demand. At this point, power has begun shifting from the intermediary to their customers. To maintain revenues, intermediaries consolidate. At some point, customers become large enough that they begin internalizing the services traditionally outsourced to intermediaries. At this juncture, the intermediaries have entered the mature phase of their lifecycles. If management has not invested in new technologies and offerings to replace their traditional business, the intermediary is acquired, merged or driven out of business. Intermediaries have to justify their existence by saving the customers money/by adding value at an attractive price. By definition, intermediary businesses are volume/economies of scale dependent.

14 PREVENTION, INTERVENTION AND TREATMENT

Profits reside where the cost of healthcare can be extracted and the savings shared.

Patients with a disease or condition can only be cured or managed by the use of pharmaceuticals, surgery, physical therapy, counseling, or medical devices that assist or replace organ function. Lifestyle changes can prevent medical conditions from materializing or getting worse. Physicians, allied health professionals and hospitals are the focal point for diagnosing, curing or managing diseases or conditions. The government and payers are the focal point for the development and promotion of lifestyle changes.

Changes in one part of the U.S. healthcare systems creates changes to other stakeholders.

The following sections concentrate on the trends driving and enabling payers, providers, pharmaceuticals and devices to grow and prosper while extracting costs from the U.S. healthcare system. While there are a myriad of other participants in the system, all are influenced and relay on this core grouping for their existence and their respective roles in delivering patient care. What happens in one part of healthcare creates changes (opportunities and/or threats) to other stakeholders. When threats or opportunities arise, stakeholders innovate to maintain or increase their market position.

The Interconnected U.S. Healthcare Enterprise

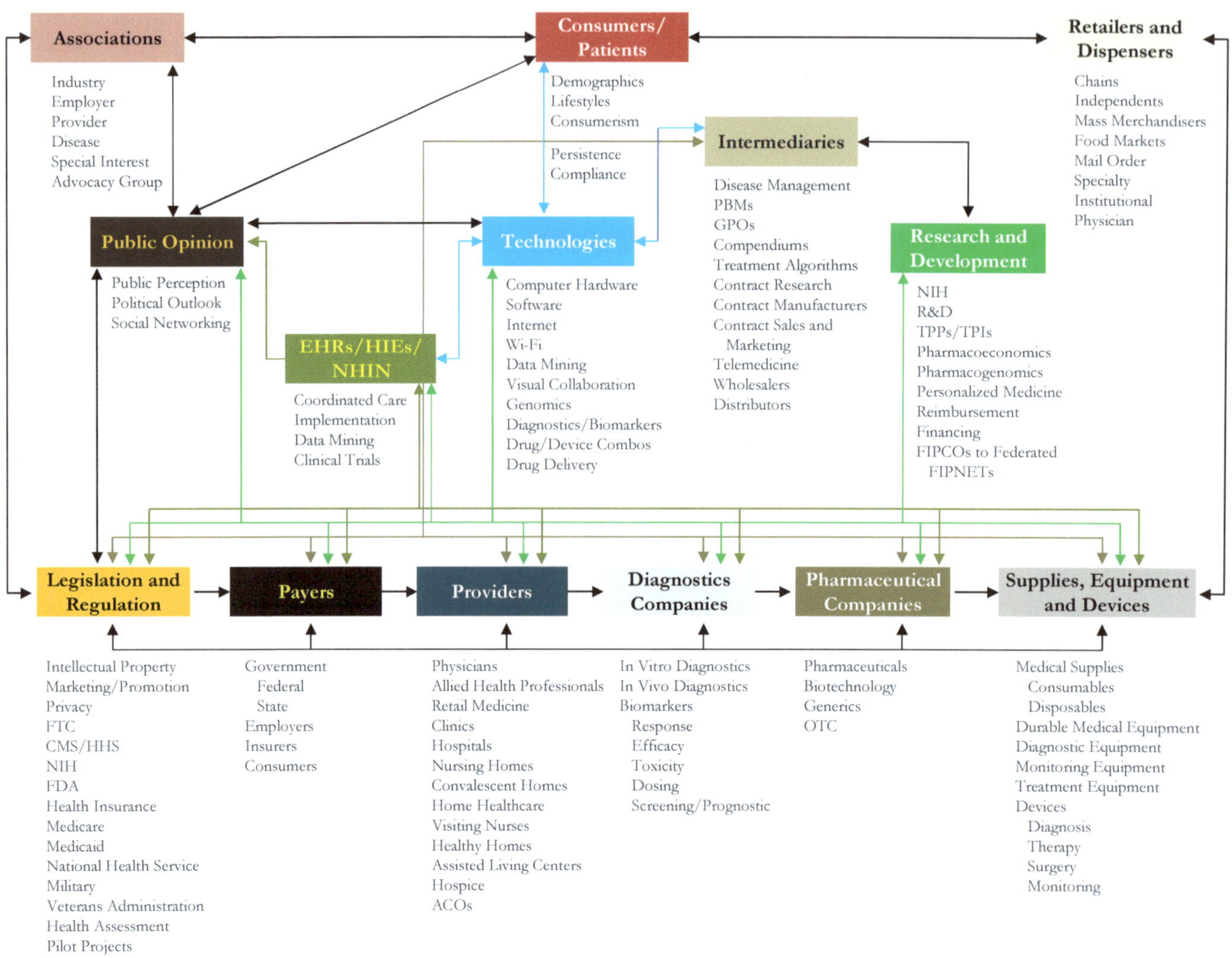

Definitions:
ACOs = Accountable Care Organizations
CMS = Centers for Medicare and Medicaid Services
FDA = Food and Drug Administration
FIPCO = Fully Integrated Pharmaceutical Company organizational structure
FIPNET = Fully Integrated Pharmaceutical Network organizational structure
FTC = Federal Trade Commission
GPOs = Group Purchasing Organizations
HHS = Department of Health and Human Services
NIH = National Institutes of Health
OTC = Over The Counter
PBMs = Pharmacy Benefit Management companies
TPI = Target Product Insert
TPP = Target Product Profile
Source: MMC International

15 HEALTH INSURANCE

Focusing on decreasing U.S. healthcare costs by insuring 32 million non-elderly uninsured by 2020.

Insuring the population has access to affordable healthcare increases utilization of preventative care, delays chronic conditions, and decreases the costs of caring for chronic conditions – increasing wellness and in turn decreasing costs. PPACA was enacted to reduce the non-elderly uninsured population by 32 million by 2020, from 19% in 2010 to about 8% of the population in 2020. It will also effect insurance coverage and where and how it is purchased. In 2009, there were 1,300+ insurance plans offered by 250 for-profit and not-for-profit U.S. health insurance companies. They provided healthcare coverage for 60% of the under 65 population and 64% of the overall U.S. population. The U.S. health insurance industry will undergo a fundamental transformation between 2012 and 2020. The potential to increase shareholder returns and create stockholder wealth is unprecedented. Success will require new strategies, competencies and organizational structures.

Enrollment By Type Of Insurance

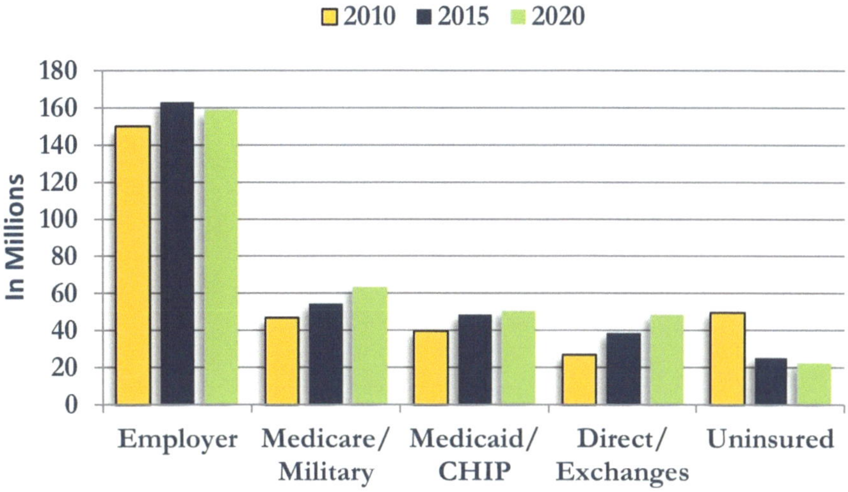

Sources: Congressional Budget Officer, 2010 Medicare Trustees Report, and MMC International analysis and projections.

The growing U.S. health insurance industry is 32% of the way to becoming a mature market.

The move towards the commoditization of health insurance will drive consolidation and the move toward market maturity throughout the 2012 to 2020 period. The top five U.S. health insurance companies, Wellpoint, United Healthcare, Aetna, Cigna and Humana are well positioned to benefit from PPACA legislation and to consolidate the U.S. healthcare industry.

U.S. Health Insurance Lifecycle

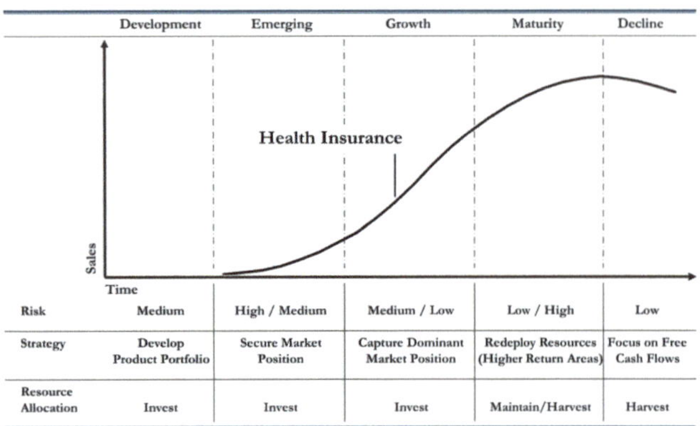

Source: MMC International

Top Five U.S. Health Insurance Companies 2009 Relative Market Shares

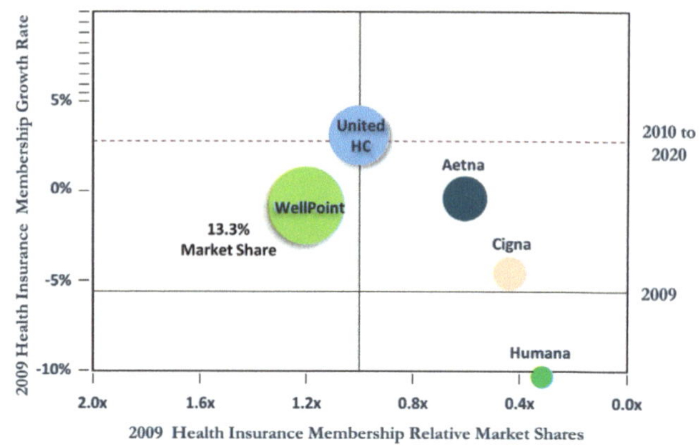

Source: MMC International

- Health insurance benefits from economies of scale.
  - There are a myriad of shared economies of scale opportunities for healthcare insurance companies.
  - State insurance regulations have protected companies from national insurance competition.
  - PPACA will result in opening cross state and national competition.
- Consolidation will require competitors to participate in all U.S. healthcare insurance market segments.
- The top five health insurers cover 41% of the insured population.
  - WellPoint, the No. 1 company, only has a 13.3% share.
- The industry is positioned for consolidation.
  - The majority of the 250 health insurance companies are state or regional companies.
- The industry leaders are well positioned to consolidate the market.

Health insurers are the best positioned to drive and profit from healthcare cost extractions.

While health insurance represents seven percent of U.S. healthcare expenditures, it will be a focus for administrative cost containment and key to health reform implementation throughout the care delivery system. Universal healthcare coverage and commoditization of health insurance will be accomplished through a number of implementation steps which began in 2010 and will go through 2016. Steps include establishment of minimum "Medical Loss Ratios" in 2011, establishing essential benefits standards, setting up insurance exchanges by 2014, an individual mandate by 2014 that requires every American to buy health insurance or pay a penalty, and changes in legislation and regulation that will allow insurance companies to sell health insurance across state lines by 2016. A key objective is to commoditize* health insurance in order to allow competition to decrease costs.

2010 U.S. Healthcare Expenditures In Billions of U.S. Dollars

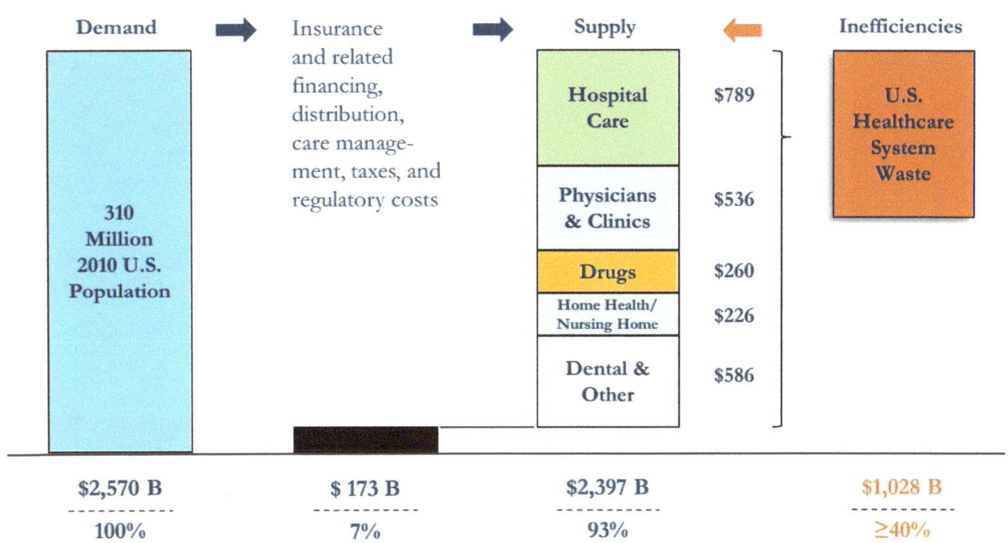

Sources: Centers for Medicare & Medicaid Services, Office of the Actuary and MMC International.

- Supply and demand equilibrium will not happen over the short term.
- Health reform will be a catalyst for market change.
- Cost-containment pressures will create a myriad of opportunities.
- Healthcare is a large, changing, and opportunity-rich marketplace.
- Actions taken by health insurers to contain cost will have ripple effects throughout the U.S. healthcare system.
- No healthcare industry participant will be left untouched.
- Cost containment represents a ≥$1 Trillion per year cost extraction opportunity.
  - Sharing in the cost savings will yield significant opportunities to increase profitability.

* Commoditization

Commoditization is the process by which goods that have economic value and are distinguishable in terms of attributes (uniqueness and/or brand) end up becoming simple commodities in the eyes of the market and consumers. It is the movement of a market from differentiated to undifferentiated price competition.

A Commodity is a good for which there is demand, but which is supplied without qualitative differentiation across a market. A commodity is equivalent no matter who produces it. Its price is determined as a function of its market as a whole. The highest price that may be charged is determined by competition. Profitability is determined by cost structure and volume.

In a perfect market, absent of intervention, competitors consolidate until it does not benefit anyone to try to increase share as the margins are equal to or less than the risk adjusted cost of capital. At this juncture, it is more attractive to invest in growth areas with higher potential returns.

Implication - The implication is that the insurance industry will consolidate over the next ten years as competitors try to secure their market positions, grow, and maintain reported profits.

The strategies followed by insurers will in part be dictated by PPACA implementing regulations.

Competitors set the maximum price that can be charged. PPACA has set the minimum "medical loss ratios". Insurers have to spend at least 80 percent of revenue on direct medical care for individual policies and 85 percent for commercial policies starting in 2011. Otherwise, they have to issue rebates to purchasers if they fail to hit the target. What is included in the definition of what is spent on direct medical care will dictate, in great part, health insurer strategies. To increase profits, insurers have to streamline and increase their economies of scale (e.g., consolidate). To succeed, insurers will: 1) position themselves for national competition (which has been enabled by PPACA), 2) move to serve all health insurance market segments, and 3) evaluate and invest in diversification opportunities. Implementation will lead to insurer consolidation and diversification.

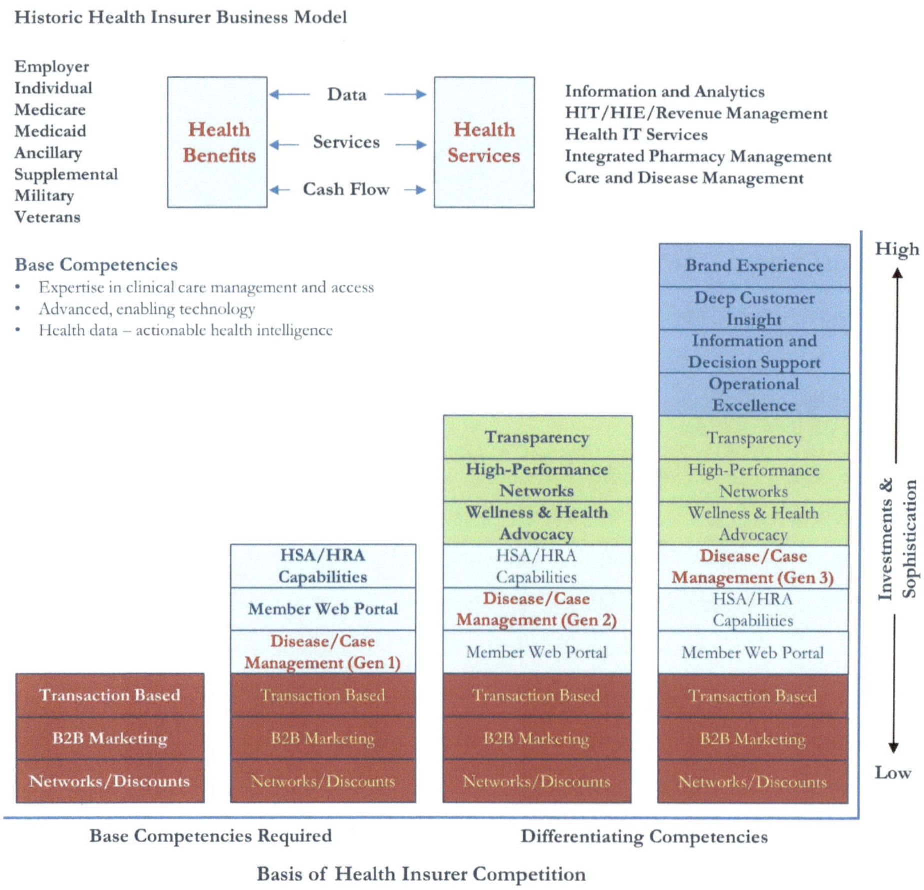

Sources: Aetna presentation; United Healthcare analyst meeting presentation; MMC International.

To succeed, health insurers will consolidate, vertically integrate, and diversify.

To succeed, insurers will: 1) position themselves for national competition, 2) move to serve all health insurance market segments, 3) vertically integrate more services (e.g., form Accountable Care Organizations, etc.), and 4) evaluate diversification opportunities. Healthcare is an opportunity rich marketplace for health insurers. Profits can be maximized by creating a number of subsidiaries under a parent company that supply services to the health insurance subsidiary that are considered inclusive in the calculation of the "medical loss ratio". The limitation is competitive pricing for similar plans.

		Complimentary Revenue/Margin Opportunities	
Market Description	**Health Insurance**	**Services**	**Delivery & Products**
	Structure, coordinate, administer, and fund health benefits	**Advancing the performance of the overall health system**	**Direct patient care and products**
Market Segments	- Individual - Employer - Medicare - Medicaid - Supplemental - Ancillary - Military and veterans	• Care management services • Technology applications and services • Data management • Consulting/actuarial/ underwriting • Banking and finance • Distribution services • PBM services	• Pharmaceutical/devices/ supplies • Physician services • Hospitals and clinics • Dialysis • Lab/testing • Etc.
Market Trends	• U.S. regulated at state and federal levels • Large market benefits from economies of scale • Consolidating market • Steady growth • Moderate margins • Exceptional cash flows	• Services to employers, consumers, care providers, life sciences, and payers • Less regulated • New markets emerging worldwide • High growth, strong margins, normal cash flows	• Majority of overall health expenditures • Domestic and international versions • Maturing and consolidating • High margins and normal cash flows

Sources: Aetna presentation; United Healthcare analyst meeting presentation; MMC International.

2011 Health Insurance Marketplace

- Medical underwriting permitted in most states
- Commissions are a significant component of individual premiums

2018 – 2020 Health Insurance Marketplace

- No medical underwriting
- Compressed rating bands
- Minimum medical loss ratios
- Competition will place a premium on brand, efficiency, service and capabilities
- Insurance exchanges

The industry will become more consolidated between 2012 and 2020 – leading to fewer but larger plans with more negotiating power.

16 PROVIDERS

Provider reimbursement, organizational structures, and care delivery will be significantly changed by 2020.

The U.S. patient care system, excluding dental care, consumed $1.6 trillion, 60 percent of 2010 U.S. healthcare expenditures. Providers are in the consolidation phase of their industry lifecycle. The U.S. patient care system is fragmented and inefficient and is where the majority of U.S. healthcare waste resides. The system requires redundant administration, information technology, accounting, facilities, support services, insurance, inventory, etc. expenditures. These duplicative costs do not contribute and may detract from patient care. Purchasing economies of scale are also constrained. Receiving care is inconvenient and time consuming for most patients. The U.S. has gone from a primary care physician and hospital centered system to a fragmented system of care. This has been driven in part by technology and physician specialization – but most of the blame can be attributed to poor legislation and implementing regulations that drove providers to segment and fragment care to maximize reimbursement. Only true marketplace competition can extract the inefficiencies from such a complex system. U.S. healthcare is a local business supported by a myriad of local, regional, national and global companies and organizations. The large number of market participants and the trillions of dollars available over the next ten years from sharing in the savings realized from eliminating waste means that this opportunity-rich marketplace will be in a period of innovation, implementation and discontinuity at least through 2020. This represents a period of significant opportunity to create corporate and personal wealth.

U.S. Patient Care Continuum

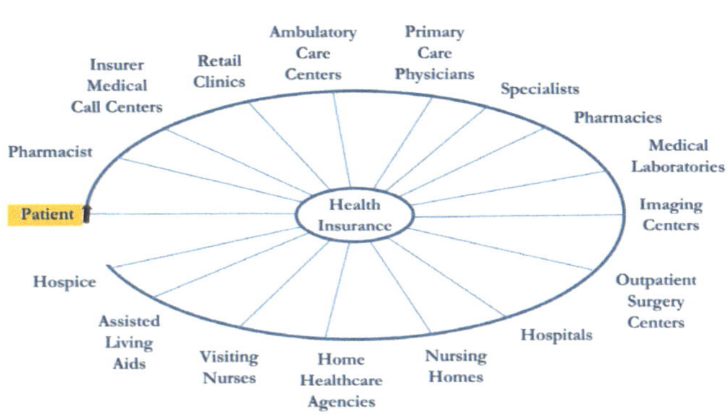

Source: MMC International

Providers

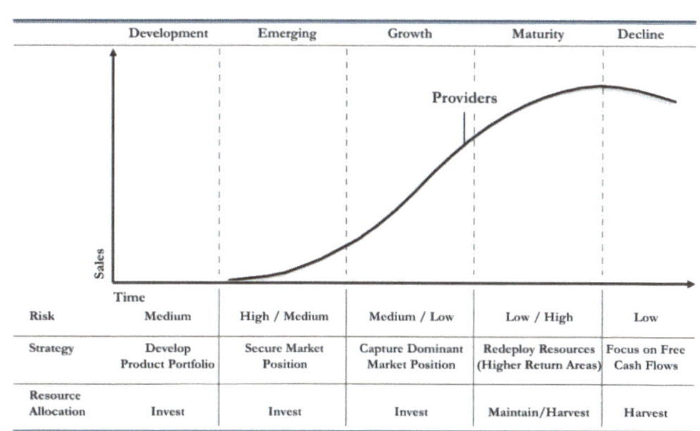

Source: MMC International

Certificate of Need (CON) requirements in effect grant monopolies and can impede system efficiencies.

The Certificate of Need (CON), in the United States, is a legal document required in many state and some federal jurisdictions before proposed acquisitions, expansions, or creations of healthcare facilities and/or services are allowed. CONs are issued by a federal or state regulatory agency with authority over an area to affirm that the plan is required to fulfill the needs of a community. A number of factors spurred states to require certificates of need in the health care industry. Chief among these was the concern that over capacity would cause competitors in an oversaturated field to cover the costs of a diluted patient pool by over-charging. This was, in part, driven by the fact that most charges were being covered by third-party payers and consumers were price insensitive. The market impact has been to de facto grant certain local monopolies. This makes it difficult to enter a CON covered market or to convince profitable entities with CON exclusivity to agree to be acquired or merged at a financially justifiable price. In a true market economy, competitors enter markets where they feel that they can profitably compete. Competition drives prices down and as a result pushes inefficient competitors out of the market. While CON laws have been repealed or not in effect in 14 states, CON laws continue in most states.

Medical Facilities And Services Regulated By Certificates Of Need
In 2010

Regulated Services	States, Districts & Commonwealth
Acute Hospital Beds	AL, AK, CT, DE, FL, GA, HI, IL, IA, KY, ME, MD, MI, MS, MO, NV, NH, NJ, NY, NC, RI, SC, TN, VT, VA, WA, WV, DC
Air Ambulance	AL, CT, ME, MA, MI, VT, DC
Ambulatory Surgical Centers (ASC)	AL, AK, CT, DE, GA, HI, IL, IA, KY, ME, MD, MA, MI, MS, MT, NV, NH, NY, NC, RI, SC, TN, VT, VA, WA, WV, DC
Burn Care	AL, CT, HI, ME, MD, NJ, NY, NC, TN, VT, WA, DC
Cardiac Catheterization	AL, AK, CT, DE, GA, HI, IL, IA, KY, ME, MD, MI, MS, MO, NH, NJ, NY, NC, RI, SC, TN, VT, VA, WA, WV, DC
Computed Tomography (CT) Scanners	AK, CT, HI, ME, MI, MO, NY, NC, RI, VT, VA, WV, DC
Gamma Knives	AL, AK, CT, GA, HI, ME, MA, MI, MS, MO, NC, RI, SC, VT, VA, DC
Home Health	AL, AR, GA, HI, KY, MD, MS, MT, NJ, NY, NC, SC, TN, VT, WA, WV, DC
Hospice	AL, AR, CT, FL, HI, KY, MD, MS, NY, NC, OR, RI, SC, TN, VT, WA, WV, DC
Intermediate Care Facilities/Mental Retardation (ICF/MR)	AR, FL, GA, HI, IL, IA, KY, LA, MD, MS, MO, MT, NV, NJ, NC, OK, SC, TN, VT, VA, WV, WI
Long Term Acute Care (LTAC)	AL, AK, CT, DE, FL, GA, HI, IL, IA, KY, ME, MD, MI, MS, MO, NH, NJ, NC, OR, RI, SC, TN, VT, VA, WA, WV, DC
Lithotripsy	AK, CT, DE, GA, HI, ME, MA, MI, MO, NY, NC, SC, TN, VT, VA, DC
Nursing Home Beds/Long-Term Care Beds	AL, AK, AR, CT, DE, FL, GA, HI, IL, IA, KY, LA, ME, MD, MA, MI, MS, MO, MT, NE, NH, NV, NJ, NY, NC, OH, OK, OR, RI, SC, TN, VT, VA, WA, WV, WI, DC
Medical Office Buildings	VT, DC
Mobile Hi Technology (CT / MRI / PET, etc)	AK, CT, HI, KY, ME, MI, MO, NH, NY, NC, RI, SC, VT, VA, WV, DC
Magnetic Resonance Imaging (MRI) Scanners	AK, CT, HI, KY, ME, MA, MI, MS, MO, NH, NY, NC, RI, SC, TN, VT, VA, WV, DC
Neo-Natal Intensive Care	AL, AK, CT, FL, GA, HI, IL, KY, ME, MD, MA, MI, NJ, NY, NC, RI, SC, TN, VT, VA, WA, WV, DC
Obstetrics Services	AL, AK, CT, GA, HI, IL, ME, MD, NY, RI, VT, VA, WA, WV, DC
Open Heart Surgery	AL, AK, CT, GA, HI, IL, IA, KY, ME, MD, MA, MI, MS, NH, NJ, NY, NC, RI, SC, TN, VT, VA, WA, WV, DC
Organ Transplants	AL, AK, CT, FL, HI, IL, IA, KY, ME, MD, MA, MI, NJ, NY, NC, RI, VT, VA, WA, WV, DC
Positron Emission Tomography (PET) Scanners	AK, CT, DE, GA, HI, KY, ME, MA, MI, MS, MO, NH, NC, RI, SC, TN, VT, VA, WV, DC
Psychiatric Services	AL, AK, AR, CT, FL, GA, HI, IL, KY, ME, MD, MA, MI, MS, NH, NJ, NC, OK, RI, SC, TN, VT, VA, WA, WV, DC
Radiation Therapy	AL, AK, CT, DE, GA, HI, IA, KY, ME, MA, MI, MS, MO, NH, NY, NC, RI, SC, TN, VT, VA, WV, DC
Rehabilitation	AL, FL, GA, HI, IL, KY, ME, MD, MA, MS, MO, MT, NE, NH, NJ, NY, NC, RI, SC, TN, VT, VA, WA, WV, DC
Renal Failure/Dialysis	AL, AK, HI, IL, ME, MS, NY, NC, VT, WA, WV, DC
Assisted Living & Residential Care Facilities	AR, LA, MO, NC, VT
Subacute Services	AK, FL, HI, IL, NC, OK, RI, SC, TN, WA, WI, VT, DC
Substance/Drug Abuse	AL, CT, FL, GA, HI, KY, ME, MD, MA, MS, MT, NH, NC, RI, SC, TN, VT, WV, DC
Swing Beds	AL, HI, IL, ME, MI, MS, MT, OR, TN, VT, WA, DC
Ultra-Sound	HI, ME, VT, DC
Other (Not otherwise covered)	AL, AR, CT, GA, IL, KY, MD, MA, MI, NC, OK, TN, WA, WI, PR

Note: According to WestLaw, September 2011, 12 states have exemptions from CON regulations called "Certificate of public advantage" : Idaho, Kansas, Louisiana, Maine, Mississippi, Montana, Nebraska, North Carolina, North Dakota, South Carolina, Tennessee, Texas, and Wisconsin.
Source: AHPA, 2010; NOTE: The categories listed above are for general information. See state-specific limitations, exceptions and requirements.

The key driver in the restructuring of providers will be changing reimbursement incentives.

In 2012, as part of PPACA, the Center for Medicare and Medicaid Services (CMS) will rework how the government pays hospitals through Medicare so facilities with better-quality treatment outcomes get higher reimbursements. This is following the lead of major insurers, such as WellPoint, the largest U.S. health insurer in terms of patients covered. Most large insurers have already begun making changes in reimbursement to tie physician payments and certain hospital payments to better outcomes. The changes are part of a broader shift within the healthcare industry to compensate health-care providers based on the quality of their care, instead of the volume of tests and treatments they perform. The entities that know how much it costs to treat a patient population, e.g., health insurers and hospitals/hospital systems that own physician groups and related healthcare services are in the best position to consolidate care, either through direct ownership and/or via a contracted network, and benefit from sharing in the cost savings. Inefficient providers will see their attractiveness/valuations wane and, absent of governmental or charitable interference, will eventually be acquired, merged or driven out of business.

WellPoint Inc. is the first major carrier to mandatorily change reimbursement for about 1,500 hospitals in 14 states that serve its Blue Cross Blue Shield plans, which cover 34 million people. Nearly 500 of WellPoint's hospitals already participate in a voluntary version of the new program which was announced in early 2011. Under the program, WellPoint is cutting off annual payment increases if the hospital fails to deliver on WellPoint's definition of quality patient care. The WellPoint formula for measuring quality of care is based 55 percent on health outcomes, 35 percent on patient-safety measures and 10 percent on patient satisfaction. It is replacing the system to help offset rising medical and other costs at hospitals. In recent years, it has raised its payments to those hospitals by an average eight percent a year. Under the new system, the company will pay increases only to hospitals that score high enough on a test based on 51 indicators of treatment quality. The indicators include whether the facility tries to prevent patients from relapsing after they leave the hospital, whether the institution follows a safety checklist, and how satisfied the hospital's patients say they are with their treatment. Facilities with poor scores will not receive a payment boost.

The change has the potential to reduce the growth in the amount WellPoint spends on inpatient care, currently about $25 billion a year, by three to five percentage points annually. Overall cost savings are expected to be greater because the new system discourages unnecessary treatments and is expected to keep people healthier.

WellPoint began testing the new approach in 2004 when it started grading hospitals on whether they created a discharge plan spelling out how patients were to take their medication and whether the facility helped plan for follow-up appointments. The changes helped reduce preventable readmissions by eight percent a year for some enrollees. One aim of the new reimbursement system is to tackle the high rate of hospital readmissions for patients who get sick again shortly after they leave the hospital/care facility. That can indicate a lapse in care. Almost one-fifth of Medicare beneficiaries who were hospitalized returned within 30 days. Preventable returns to the hospital cost WellPoint $2 billion a year.

Almost 500 of WellPoint's hospitals already participating in its voluntary version of the new program are getting average pay increases of seven to nine percent a year. When a hospital renews its contract with WellPoint, it will be required to report quality benchmarks to qualify for a rate increase. University of Virginia Health System in Charlottesville, a participant in the original program, received an extra $2 million from WellPoint because it racked up a good quality score. The new system serves as an incentive to enhance patient safety, rather than being punitive for not meeting it.

Health insurer competition will drive cost extractions from the provider system.

Patient/consumer shopping for quality care at a competitive price will drive quality improvements.

On May 2, 2011 the Department of Health and Human Services (HHS) announced the Hospital Value-Based Purchasing Program, created under PPACA. In fiscal year (FY) 2013, the Hospital Value-Based Purchasing Program will distribute an estimated $850 million in incentive payments to hospitals based on their overall performance on a set of quality measures that have been linked to improved clinical processes of care and patient satisfaction. The new program encourages hospitals to adopt practices that have been shown to be effective in improving patient outcomes. Equally important, it will be looking very carefully at whether the patient feels that he or she has been treated with respect and compassion, and has been given the opportunity to participate in decisions about treatment. To insure transparency, patients/consumers are now able to compare how their hospital measures up on 44 different care quality measures by going to www.HealthCare.gov/compare. Consumers can also see how nursing homes, home healthcare agencies and dialysis centers compare on certain quality measures. This engages the consumers by allowing them to distinguish adequate care from excellent care. It encourages hospital shopping and pressures local hospitals to focus on quality of care and patient satisfaction or risk losing patients/revenues. While the information is more limited on nursing homes, home healthcare agencies, and dialysis centers, the information on the site also engages consumers – driving these providers to focus on quality of care and patient satisfaction. Providers that fail to adapt will underperform and as a direct result suffer decreasing valuations - absent of government or charitable intervention, they will be acquired, merged or driven out of business.

The hospital incentive payments ($850 million in FY 2013) will be taken from what Medicare, the largest payer for hospital services, otherwise would have spent for hospital stays. The size of the fund will gradually increase over time, resulting in a shift from payments based on volume to payments based on performance/quality of care. This redirection will encourage care quality improvements and is intended to result in significant, additional savings to Medicare, taxpayers, and enrollees over time. This is expected to help improve the odds that every patient receives the best care, regardless of the location of treatment. It also encourages "patient-centered" care. The Hospital Value-Based Purchasing Program captures information about patient satisfaction with their care. It asks the important questions about how well hospital staff communicated with patients during and after a hospitalization and the overall cleanliness of the hospital environment. The results for each hospital are posted on www.HealthCare.gov/compare. The website provides tools that facilitate comparison of up to three hospitals, thereby enabling consumer choice. These efforts complement efforts by health insurance companies and should benefit all patients.

Various care management models and organizational structures will materialize.

The opportunities are so vast and the marketplace is so complex that a myriad of reimbursement, organizational and management models will materialize between 2012 and 2020 to more cost-effectively deliver an improved quality of care as measured by patient outcomes. PPACA legislation contains a number of reimbursement provisions to promote more efficient integrated care. They include reimbursement programs, incentives, pilot programs, etc. Implementing regulations will play a significant role in how the new organizations are developed and their speed of adoption and implementation. What is clear is that health insurers, hospital groups/hospitals, and physician group practices can organize into Accountable Care Organizations (ACOs) and participate and financially benefit from these programs. Healthcare delivery is a local business. As such, solutions will materialize on a catchment area by catchment area basis.

2010 Level of Integration

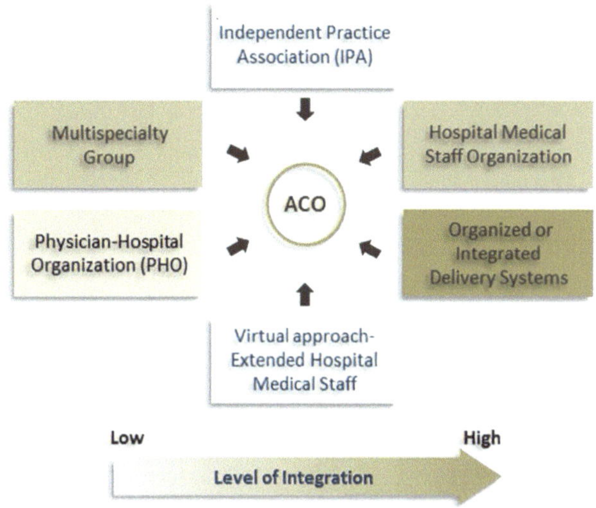

Adapted From: What are Accountable Care Organizations?, Healthcare Economist, January 26, 2010.

PPACA calls for implementation of payment reform pilots and implementation from 2011 through 2015. However, implementation will go well beyond 2015.

2011

- The Health and Human Services (HHS) secretary created the Center for Medicare and Medicaid Innovation to test both payment and healthcare delivery techniques.
- Annual increases in hospital payments will begin to be limited to account for productivity gains.

2012

- Providers that qualify as accountable-care organizations (ACOs) are to share in cost savings they achieve for Medicare.
- The HHS secretary is to establish a demonstration program to test payment incentives for home-based primary care.
- Medicare payments to hospitals are to be reduced to account for preventable hospital readmissions.
- On Oct. 1, hospitals that meet certain performance standards are to become eligible for value-based incentive payments allotted by fiscal year.
- The HHS secretary is to adjust the Medicare physician fee schedule to reflect variety in operating expenses for medical practices in different geographic areas.
- High-quality Medicare Advantage plans are to begin receiving bonus payments.

2013

- The HHS secretary is to establish a Medicare pilot program to evaluate bundled payments for episodes of care.

2015

- On Jan. 1, 2015, the Center for Medicare and Medicaid Services (CMS) will begin using the Medicare fee schedule to give larger payments to physicians who provide high-quality care compared with cost.

Physicians are moving from private practices to group and hospital physician practices.

Physician services represented about $532 billion, 20.9 percent, of the $2.6 Trillion spent in 2010 on U.S. healthcare expenditures. About 32 percent of the 592,410 physicians practicing in the United States in 2010 were in solo or two-physician private practices. This number is forecast to continue to decrease because physicians are increasingly willing to give up autonomy in trade for less administrative requirements, an ability to concentrate on patient care, predictable compensation, and a better quality of life. According to data released June 3, 2010, by the Medical Group Management Association, 65 percent of established physicians hired, and 49 percent of those finishing residencies, landed positions in hospital-based practices in 2009. Community-based physicians, previously in private groups, are increasingly selling their practices or seeking employment directly with healthcare systems and hospitals.

U.S. Physicians By Type Of Practice

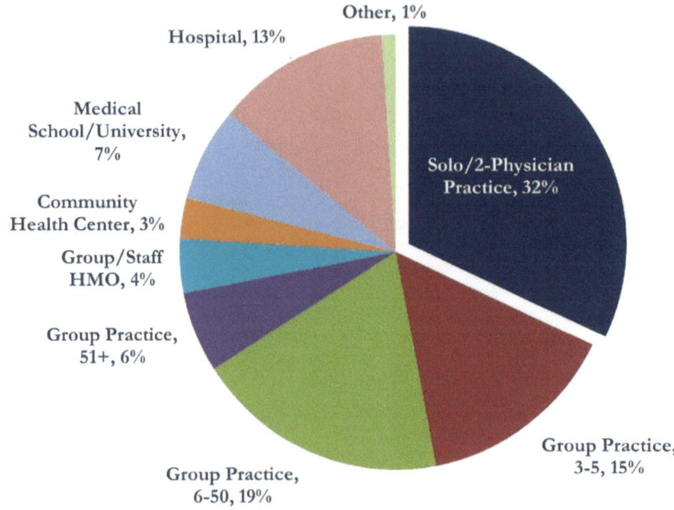

Source: HSC 2008 Health Tracking Physician Survey.

2011 Top Twenty United States Medical Groups
By Number of Physicians

Rank	Medical Group	Headquarters	State	Offices	Physicians
1	Kaiser Permanente Medical Group	Santa Clara	CA	374	8,890
2	Mayo Clinic	Jacksonville	FL	32	1,769
3	Montefiore Medical Center-RAD	Bronx	NY	448	1,594
4	Cleveland Clinic	Cleveland	OH	80	1,331
5	Presbyterian Medical Group	Albuquerque	NM	421	1,030
6	Lakeside Medical Associates	Mission Hills	CA	501	927
7	Palo Alto Medical	Clinic Santa Cruz	CA	37	907
8	Novant Medical Group	Winston Salem	NC	253	883
9	University Pittsburgh Physicians	Pittsburgh	PA	86	870
10	Henry Ford Medical Group	Detroit	MI	66	864
11	EmCare Nationwide	Las Vegas	NV	158	824
12	Carolinas Physicians Network	Charlotte	NC	158	804
13	Intermountain Medical Group	Salt Lake City	UT	139	751
14	Iowa Health Physicians Pediatrics	Cedar Rapids	IA	263	733
15	Emory Clinic	Atlanta	GA	103	729
16	Scott & White Clinic	Temple	TX	45	706
17	Fairview Physician Associates	Minneapolis	MN	120	696
18	Allina Medical Clinic	Minneapolis	MN	52	685
19	Marshfield Clinic	Marshfield	WI	38	671
20	UC Davis Medical Group	Roseville	CA	57	670

Source: SK&A, A Cegedim Company.

Physician compensation is moving toward compensating for patient care rather than procedures.

This trend of physicians becoming employees of hospitals and groups is being complemented by changes in physician compensation practices. Medical institutions have learned from past mistakes. Rather than pay fixed salaries, they are increasingly utilizing productivity-based compensation formulas designed to make physicians happier, more productive and to assist the institution to reach certain strategic goals/benchmarks of quality and patient satisfaction, i.e., to align physician compensation with the institution's goals and objectives. Physicians have also learned from prior mistakes, e.g., the collapse of physician practice management companies (PPMs) which flourished and then lost their value in the 1990s. Numerous physician-led alignment models serve as alternatives to direct employment of doctors by hospitals. Examples include the physician-hospital organization (PHO), the independent practice association (IPA), physician practice management groups, a potentially reemerging PPM sector, and accountable care organizations (ACOs). ACOs, which are touted in PPACA, allow collective contracting without the need for employment by a single entity. Proliferation of these models could preserve physicians' independence. Regardless, the trend will be to fewer independent physicians as older physicians that had been in solo or two physician practices are reaching retirement age. This trend also means that demand for physicians' assistants and nurse practitioners will persist as hospitals and large group practices are increasingly utilizing them as physician extenders to increase physician productivity and group and/or hospital reimbursement/profitability.

Efforts to change physician compensation began long before the March 23, 2010 implementation of PPACA. It has been driven by demands from large employers, such as IBM, and health insurers. United Healthcare (the nation's second largest health insurer) is moving away from paying doctors solely on the basis of how many services they provide, and will start rewarding them for the overall quality of care patients receive. This accommodates using physician extenders, e.g., physician's assistants and/or nurse practitioners to meet the measurable patient quality matrixes. The theory is that by providing a home base for patients and coordinating their treatment, doctors can improve care, prevent unnecessary emergency room visits, reduce hospitalizations, and lower overall medical spending. As an example, in 2009, United Healthcare and IBM began testing a "Medical Home" new model of healthcare (a model encouraged by PPACA) that will give doctors more authority and money than usual in return for closely monitoring their patients' progress, even when patients go to specialists or require hospitalization.

Cost of care per day is least expensive for home healthcare, most expensive for hospital care.

The least expensive care, outside of self-care directed by a physician and supported by family and or friends, is assisted living, followed by home healthcare services supplied by home healthcare agencies, and then skilled nursing homes. The most intensive and costly care is proved by hospitals. Hospitals, nursing homes and home healthcare are the traditional central organizations around which care is delivered. Utilization is significantly impacted by Medicare, Medicaid, other government and third-party reimbursement. For most patients, the ideal recuperative setting is home.

Comparison of Hospital, Skilled Nursing Facility, and Home Healthcare Medical Charges 2005 to 2009

	2005	2006	2007	2008	2009
Hospital (Per Day)	$4,999	$5,475	$5,895	$6,196	$6,200
Skilled Nursing Home (Per Day)	504	519	558	590	622
Home Healthcare (Per Visit)	125	129	130	134	135

Source: *Basic Statistics About Home Care, Updated 2010* by The National Association for Home Care & Hospice.

The average American hospital barely breaks even.

There were 5,232 hospitals in 2009, an increase of 84 hospitals over 2008. In 2010, hospitals accounted for about 30 percent, $789 billion, of U.S. healthcare expenditures - more than physicians, nursing homes and home healthcare expenditures combined. The average American hospital barely breaks even. In 2009, 16.9 percent of hospitals were for-profit, 59.7 percent were not-for-profit, and 23.4 percent were government owned. The median operating margin for 200-bed hospitals and above was slightly negative (-0.7%) in 2009. Uncompensated care has been relatively stable at six percent of hospital costs for many years, despite a steady increase in the percentage of people uninsured. The individual mandate contained in PPACA requires every American to have health insurance by 2014 or pay a penalty. This provision (which is being aggressively challenged by Republicans) is expected to decrease hospital costs for uncompensated care, move most hospitals into the black, and unleash funds that would allow investments in staff, equipment, systems, processes and facilities to improve efficiencies and the quality of care. Patient satisfaction scores have been found to correlate meaningfully with profitability. Industry experts argue that hospitals become more profitable by delivering higher quality care. Moody's, the credit rating service, now looks closely at hospital clinical quality measures when rating debt offerings. Moody's argues that a strategy aimed at quality can result in improved market share, better ability to recruit and retain physicians, lower nursing vacancy/turnover rates; and thereby improve financial performance. The hospital industry is on its way to capitalizing on the ability to increase profits by improving care while extracting costs. Hospitals have been quietly consolidating into multiple hospital systems (MHS) in recent years. Now many hospital "systems" dominate their regional markets. This allows them more negotiating leverage with payers.

Number of U.S. Hospitals In and Out of Multihospital Systems (MHS), 2001-2009

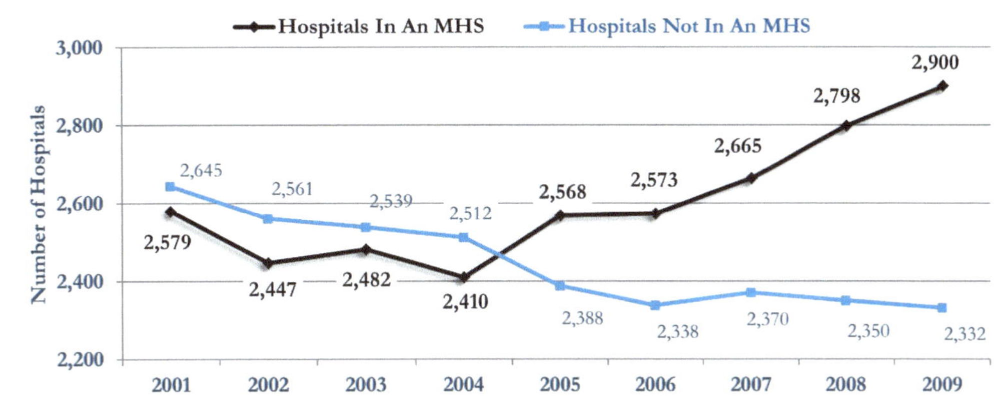

	2001	2002	2003	2004	2005	2006	2007	2008	2009
Total Hospitals:	5,224	5,008	5,021	4,922	4,956	4,911	5,035	5,148	5,232
% In An MHS	49.4%				51.8%				55.4%

Data Sources: Prepared by MMC International from SDI 2011 data and sanofi-aventis Managed Care Digest Series/Hospitals/Systems Digest 2011-2012 chart.

Some hospitals, which includes not-for-profit hospitals, are very profitable.

There is a growing gap between the have and have-not hospitals. An analysis done by Forbes magazine of the American Hospital Directory (which is based on operating income figures that hospitals must report to the federal Medicare program each year) found 24 hospitals with over 200 beds making an operating margin of 25 percent or more. That compares favorably to the most successful drug companies and exceeds General Electric's 13.6 percent 2010 operating margin. Fifteen of the 25 hospitals were part of for-profit chains. HCA, the largest hospital system in the United States, had 10 hospitals in the top 25. Big non-profits that made the list included Mayo Clinic's main hospitals and Ohio State University's hospital. For hospitals to be economically viable in the future, they will have to align performance and payment systems to meet quality and efficiency-related goals; use process-improvement tools to increase efficiency and reduce costs; pursue coverage options to ensure patient access to, and affordability of, healthcare services; and address how both general acute care hospitals and specialty hospitals can cost competitively deliver quality healthcare. A key component in the future will be the ability to keep costs in line with those of the most efficient multihospital systems. If they are not able to compete and are subjected to marketplace competition, their valuations will decrease and they will be acquired, merged or driven out of business.

Total Costs Per Admission, By MHS Ownership, 1999-2009

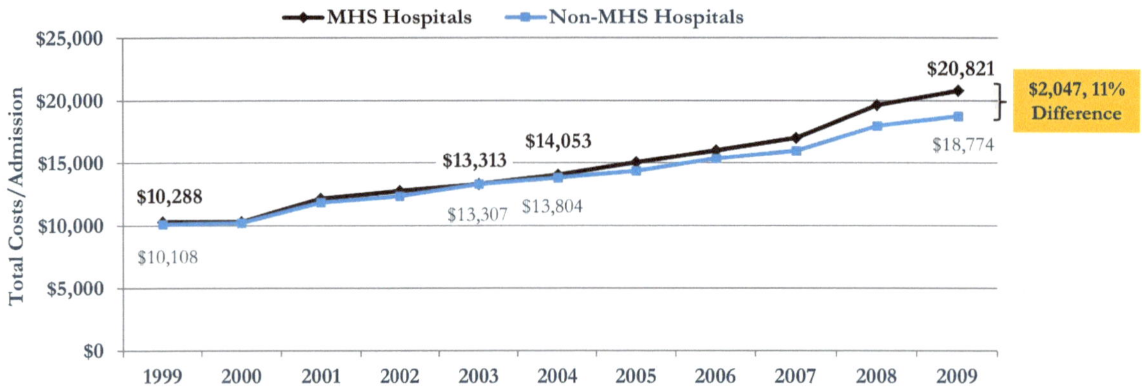

Data Sources: SDI 2011 data and sanofi-aventis Managed Care Digest Series/Hospitals/Systems Digest 2011-2012.

Top 20 Multihospital Systems Ranked By Number of Staffed Beds

Rank By Number of Beds	Multihospital System	Headquarters	Number of Hospitals Owned 2008	2009
	For Profit			
1	HCA	Nashville, TN	156	156
2	Community Health Systems	Brentwood, TN	119	123
3	Tenet Health System	Dallas, TX	52	49
7	Health Management Associates	Naples, FL	61	61
15	Universal Health Services	King of Prussia, PA	22	23
17	LifePoint Hospitals, Inc.	Brentwood, TN	49	53
20	Vanguard Health Systems	Nashville, TN	15	17
	Not-For-Profit			
4	Ascension Health	Saint Louis, MO	51	53
5	Catholic Healthcare West	San Francisco, CA	38	38
6	Catholic Health Initiatives	Denver, CO	70	67
8	Kaiser Permanente	Oakland, CA	34	35
9	Trinity Health	Novi, MI	30	32
10	Adventist Health System	Winter Park, FL	35	35
11	Providence Health and Services	Renton, WA	25	25
12	North Shore–Long Island Jewish Health System	Great Neck, NY	10	13
13	Sutter Health	Sacramento, CA	31	30
14	Catholic Health East	Newtown Square, PA	19	19
16	CHRISTUS Health	Irving, TX	23	22
18	Catholic Health Partners	Cincinnati, OH	30	31
	Government			
19	New York City Health and Hospitals Corporation	New York, NY	9	11
	Total Hospitals Owned by Top 20 MHSs		**879**	**893**
	% of Total U.S. Hospitals		**17.1%**	**17.1%**

Data Sources: Slide and table prepared by MMC International from SDI 2011 data and sanofi-aventis Managed Care Digest Series/Hospitals/Systems Digest 2011-2012.

The trend is towards highly integrated healthcare systems to increase negotiating power with payers.

The number of hospitals in highly integrated systems have increased 22.3 percent in seven years - from 1,778 hospitals, 35.4 percent of all hospitals in 2004, to 2,175 hospitals, 41.6 percent of all hospitals in 2010. The trend clearly is toward the integration of hospitals into highly integrated healthcare systems. In 2010, there were 335 highly integrated healthcare systems. These systems either own or contract with at least three components of healthcare delivery, including at least one acute-care hospital, at least one physician component, and at least one other component of care. Highly integrated healthcare systems also have at least one system wide contract with a payer. These organizations, through ownership or formal agreements, align healthcare facilities in order to deliver integrated healthcare services by improving quality and reducing costs to a defined geographical area. They have been formed to market themselves as one unit to payers.

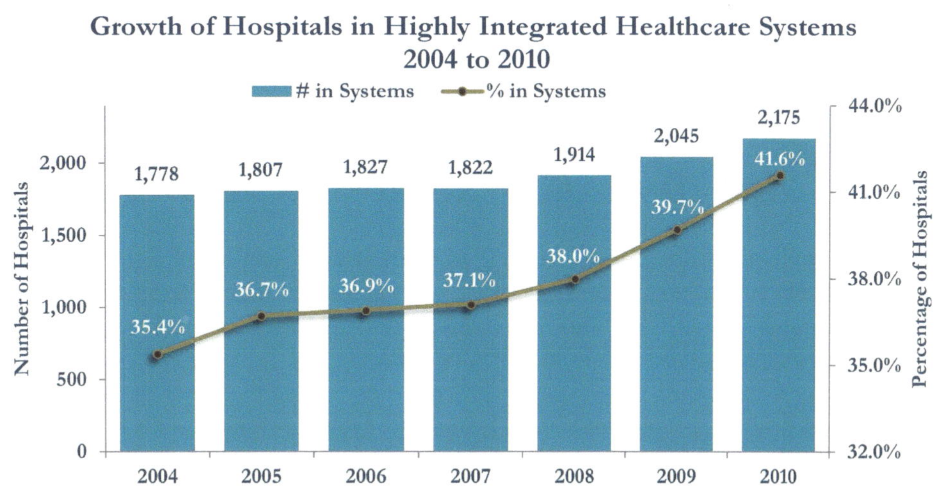

Sources: Adapted by MMC International from SDI 2011 data and sanofi-aventis *Managed Care Digest Series/Hospitals/Systems Digest 2011-2012.*

20 Selected Integrated Systems and Their Facilities

Integrated Health System	Headquarters Location	# of Owned/ Affiliated Managed Care Organizations		# of Licensed Hospitals		# of Licensed Nursing Homess		# of Licensed Home Healthcare Agencies		# of Medical Group Practices	
		2008	2009	2008	2009	2008	2009	2008	2009	2008	2009
Advocate Health Care	Oak Brook, IL	0	0	9	11	0	0	9	7	35	35
Allina Hospitals and Clinics	Minneapolis, MN	0	0	16	16	1	1	1	0	42	41
Banner Health	Phoenix, AZ	1	1	22	22	4	4	4	3	17	17
Baylor Health Care System	Dallas, TX	0	0	20	21	1	1	1	1	16	16
BJC HealthCare	Saint Louis, MO	0	0	12	12	3	3	5	4	6	6
Carle Foundation Hospital	Urbana, IL	1	1	1	1	2	3	1	1	7	15
Carolinas HealthCare System	Charlotte, NC	1	1	23	23	7	9	7	6	48	47
Department of Health Services	Los Angeles, CA	1	1	4	4	0	0	0	0	38	38
Detroit Medical Center	Detroit, MI	1	1	8	8	0	0	0	0	0	0
Geisinger Health System	Danville, PA	1	1	4	4	0	0	0	1	33	32
HCA Houston Division	Houston, TX	0	0	16	15	0	0	0	0	0	0
Henry Ford Health System	Detroit, MI	1	1	8	8	2	2	4	2	29	28
Legacy Health System	Portland, OR	1	1	5	5	0	0	0	0	5	5
Ministry Health Care	Milwaukee, WI	1	1	15	15	0	0	7	8	6	6
Presbyterian Healthcare Services	Albuquerque, NM	1	1	7	7	1	1	2	2	15	15
Sentara Healthcare	Norfolk, VA	4	3	8	9	7	7	7	6	20	20
Sharp HealthCare	San Diego, CA	1	1	7	7	3	2	1	1	17	14
Sutter Health	Sacramento, CA	1	0	35	34	1	1	15	15	45	44
Temple University Health System	Philadelphia, PA	0	0	4	3	0	0	1	1	1	1
Tenet South Florida Health System	Fort Lauderdale, FL	0	0	11	11	0	0	0	0	0	0

Source: sanofi-aventis *Managed Care Digest Series/Hospitals/Systems 2011-2012* and SDI.

Highly integrated healthcare systems are getting bigger and vertically integrating care.

The 335 highly integrated healthcare systems owned or contracted with 23,246 provider units in 2010. The growth in integrated systems has come from the systems adding more provider units and becoming larger. Provider units include healthcare facilities such as hospitals, health maintenance organizations (HMOs), nursing homes, home health agencies, physician practices and medical groups, diagnostic imaging centers and freestanding outpatient surgery centers. Each highly integrated healthcare system either contracts with or owns at least three of these facility types. However, such a healthcare facility is not necessarily affiliated with only one integrated system; it may contract with or be owned in part by more than one integrated system. Each such relationship is counted as a "provider unit" of the system with which it is affiliated. In accordance, the total number of provider units is greater than the total number of healthcare facilities affiliated with highly integrated healthcare systems. Since 2001, the number of highly integrated healthcare systems with 21 or more provider units increased by 25 percent, from 195 systems in 2001 to 244 in 2010. The strategy is to move to owned from contracted provider units and to extract costs by vertically integrating. By focusing efforts on specific catchment areas, the systems position themselves to better negotiate with payers as they control a significant number of covered lives in a specific geographic area. The highly integrated healthcare systems are positioned to extract costs by applying organizational structure efficiencies, improving coordinated care by leveraging information technology investments, negotiating better prices through centralized purchasing, and controlling quality and outcomes through outcomes-based incentive compensation. They are also able to create a brand image in patients' minds which allows them to charge competitive prices for their services. In turn, they position themselves to earn the maximum profit sharing incentives from delivering higher quality cost-competitive/effective care. Vertical integration is the trend for providers. It extracts costs which are not directly related to patient care and allow better negotiating leverage with payers and suppliers. Successful systems will make high returns when compared to the norm. The period from 2012 to 2020 will be one of discontinuities, experimentation, implementation, and consolidation. It will unleash and create wealth for efficiently run providers and their stakeholders/stockholders.

Growth In Owned and Contracted Provider Units In Highly Integrated Healthcare Systems
2001 versus 2010

	Number Contracted				Number Owned				Total			
FACILITY TYPE	2001	2010	% Change	Growth	2001	2010	% Change	Growth	2001	2010	% Change	Growth
Physician Practice (1)	2,394	3,178	32.70%		3,747	7,713	105.80%		6,141	10,891	77.30%	
Hospitals (2)	891	716	−19.6 %		1,316	1,921	46.0%		2,207	2,637	19.5%	
Home Health Agency	345	198	−42.6%		350	406	16.0%		695	604	−13.1%	
Nursing Home	252	343	36.1%		257	474	84.4%		509	817	60.5%	
Freestanding Outpatient Surgery Center	138	183	32.6%		178	470	164.0%		316	653	106.6%	
HMO/PPO	52	36	−30.8%		103	120	16.5%		155	156	0.6%	
Rehabilitation Center	194	197	1.5%		311	348	11.9%		505	545	7.9%	
Diagnostic Imaging Center	150	146	−2.7%		170	1,049	517.1%		320	1,195	273.4%	
Hospice	79	47	−40.5%		52	90	73.1%		131	137	4.6%	
Mental Health Center	61	58	−4.9%		75	113	50.7%		136	171	25.7%	
Dialysis Center	43	92	114.0%		63	88	39.7%		106	180	69.8%	
Cancer Center	41	116	182.9%		61	439	619.7%		102	555	444.1%	
Other	736	1,798	144.3%		908	2,907	220.2%		1,644	4,705	186.2%	
TOTAL	5,376	7,108	32.20%		7,591	16,138	112.60%		12,967	23,246	79.30%	

Sources: Prepared by MMC International from sanofi-aventis Managed Care Digest Series® Hospitals/Systems Digest 2011-2012 and SDI data.

The total number of provider units grew 79.3 percent between 2001 and 2010 to 23,246. The growing trends shows that a shift is occurring in the marketplace from contracted to owned units. The number of owned units grew at 112.6 percent to 16,138 versus a growth of 32.2 percent for contracted units. Another key trend was investments in highly profitable specialty centers such as cancer centers (owned units increased 620 percent from 61 in 2001 to 439 in 2010) and diagnostic imaging (owned units increased 517 percent from 170 in 2001 to 1,049 in 2010). The focus appears to be on services portfolio management which will allow these systems to earn higher returns than their local competitors. This will drive up their valuations while depressing competitor acquisition prices. This position the highly integrated systems to further consolidate their local positions, absent of government intervention, by acquiring or taking control of inefficient local providers – further leveraging their existing investments and reinforcing their negotiating position with both suppliers and payers. This process will extract inefficiencies/costs, improve overall care quality, and position the system to share in the cost savings.

A number of alternatives exist for non-hospital patient care. Cost and reimbursement drive demand.

The least expensive patient care is self-care at home under medical professional direction. Smart equipment and devices will allow more patients to continue independent living. Technology will transform where and how patients are managed and treated. The alternatives in broad groupings include: 1) Assisted Living, 2) Assisted Living, Dementia Care, 3) Congregate Housing, 4) Continuing Care Retirement Community, 5) Independent Living, and Nursing Homes.

Assisted Living is a long-term care option that combines housing, support services and health care, as needed. Assisted living is designed for individuals who require assistance with everyday activities such as meals, medication management or assistance, bathing, dressing and transportation. Some residents may have memory disorders including Alzheimer's, or they may need help with mobility, incontinence or other challenges.

Assisted Living, Dementia Care are for individuals with Alzheimer's disease or related dementia. They are often referred to as "Special Care Units (SCUs)." Often, they are housed in a special wing of the assisted living community with additional security, cueing devices and other specific architectural features. These areas are state licensed and provide programming specific to the population being served. They are staffed with individuals who are specifically trained to work with individuals who have some form of dementia. SCUs can differ in the level of care they provide along the continuum of the disease. For instance, some assisted living communities will accept individuals with Alzheimer's or related dementia through the entire disease process whereas other will only accept individuals who are in the early stage of the disease.

Congregate Housing is similar to independent living except that it usually provides convenience or supportive services like meals, housekeeping, and transportation in addition to rental housing.

Continuing Care Retirement Community is a community that offers several levels of assistance, including independent living, assisted living and nursing home care. It is different from other housing and care options for seniors because it usually provides a written agreement or long-term contract between the resident (frequently lasting the term of the resident's lifetime) and the community, which offers a continuum of housing, services and health care system, commonly all on one campus or site. They are paid for through long-term contracts with the residents. They are covered by state regulations in 38 states and are usually classified as an insurance model governed by the state department of insurance or another similar entity. Each part of the community may be subject to separate oversight. For example, housing could be regulated at the local level, assisted living regulated at the state level, and the nursing home part of the community governed by state and federal regulations.

Independent Living is designed for seniors who require little or no assistance with the activities of daily living. Independent living units provide services for residents such as housekeeping, laundry and meals. Residents of independent units may have some home health care services provided by in-house staff or an outside agency. These residents pay a rental rate or monthly fee. The residential living setting for senior adults may or may not provide hospitality or supportive services. Under this living arrangement, the senior adult leads an independent lifestyle that requires minimal or no extra assistance. Generally referred to as elderly housing in the government-subsidized environment, independent living also includes rental assisted or market rate apartments or cottages where residents usually have complete choice in whether to participate in the community's services or programs.

Nursing Homes are medical care options that provide nursing or convalescent care for three or more persons unrelated to the licensee. A nursing home provides care of chronic conditions or short-term convalescent or rehabilitative care, for which medical and nursing care are indicated. Some residents are admitted for short stays of convalescent or rehabilitative care following hospitalization. In addition to licensure, nursing homes that wish to receive Medicare and Medicaid reimbursement must be certified in accordance with federal law. Beyond licensure and certification requirements, nursing homes must also honor the federal Nursing Home Patient's Bill of Rights. These rights are designed to promote and protect the well-being of nursing home residents. Funding options for nursing home care include: private funding, long-term care insurance, Medicare, and in large part Medicaid. Paying for nursing home care is a major concern for many families as well as the government. Historically, Medicaid has paid for about half of the total cost of nursing home care, with Medicare and private long-term care insurance paying but a fraction of the cost.

There were 20,858 Senior Living Providers and Nursing Homes that provided nursing care in 2011.

There were an estimated 20,858 facilities in the United States in May 2011 that provided nursing care. These can be broadly segmented into "Senior Living Providers" and "Nursing Homes". Senior Living Providers include Assisted Living (including developmentally disabled), Independent Living (includes Board and Care), Continuing Care (includes Retired Living and Residential), and Memory Care (includes resident and adult day care) facilities/communities. Nursing Homes include Skilled Nursing, Personal Care, Rehab, Nursing and Hospice facilities. Skilled Nursing represented 66 percent of facilities followed by Assisted Living which accounted for 13 percent. Seventy-six percent of all facilities were represented by traditional nursing homes. Almost half of the facilities are privately owned, leaving room for consolidation. Groups own 45 percent; and the government owns about five percent.

Percent of Nursing Care Facilities By Type

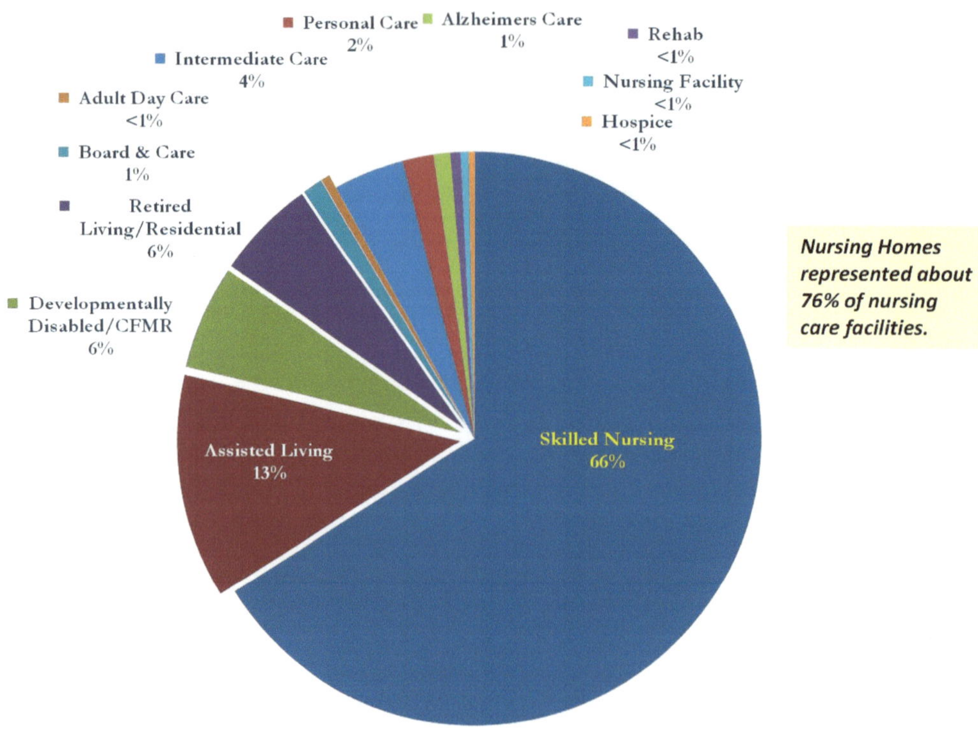

Source: MMC International and SK&A data.

Nursing Facility Ownership

Type of Ownership	Number of Facilities	Percent of Facilities
Privately Owned	10,369	49.7%
Group Owned	9,476	45.4%
Federal Government Owned	627	3.0%
City Owned	37	0.2%
County Owned	290	1.4%
State Owned	59	0.3%
Total	20,858	100.0%

Source: SK&A.

Senior Living Providers are in the growth phase of their industry lifecycle.

There are approximately 5,000 senior living facilities in the United States. This is far from a consolidated industry. The company that owns the most facilities, Brookdale Senior Living, had 557 properties, around 10 percent of total properties. Demand for Senior Living Providers will be fueled nationally by a more affluent aging population and changing care reimbursement practices. Lack of financing has resulted in a slowdown in construction of senior living facilities which allowed the sector an opportunity to catch up with demand. It also resulted in the consolidation of weaker competitors by cash rich REITs (Real Estate Investment Trusts) and groups like Blackstone Real Estate Advisors, the world leader in private equity real estate investment. The limited amount of available acquisition targets/mega-deals has led to higher valuations. Historically, increased valuations attract development and construction capital for new facilities. Senior Living Providers are in the growth phase of their industry Lifecycle. However, markets are local, meaning that some markets may be saturated; many are balanced, while others have pent up demand. Most of the facilities are privately owned. The value of the market has been validated as more private equity and REITs are investing in senior living facilities.

Senior Living Providers Lifecycle

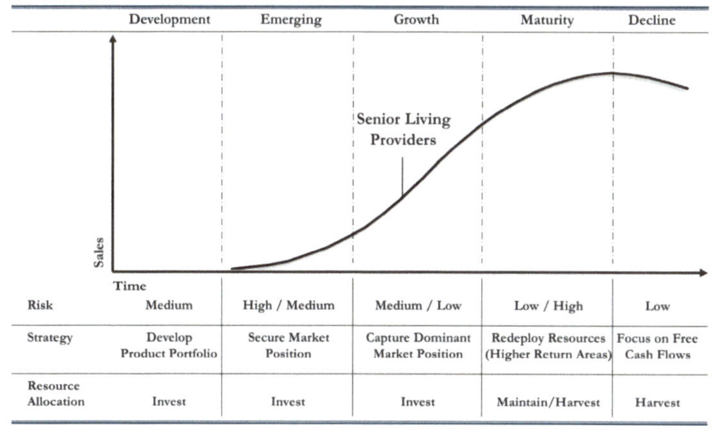

Source: MMC International.

Top 20 Largest Senior Living Providers (January 1, 2011)

		Resident Capacity (Some Units Dually Licensed)					
Rank	Company	Total	Assisted Living	Independent Living	Memory Care	Total No. Of Properties	Public or Private
1	Emeritus Senior Living	51,725	46,777	4,948	6,680	484	**Public**
2	Brookdale Senior Living	47,986	27,568	20,418	3,205	557	**Public**
3	Holiday Retirement	36,863	309	36,554	-	313	*Private*
4	Sunrise Senior Living	33,983	28,131	5,852	8,418	319	**Public**
5	Life Care Services, LLC	25,963	4,650	21,313	1,047	85	*Private*
6	Five Star Senior Living	16,870	10,489	6,381	2,423	177	**Public**
7	Horizon Bay Retirement	15,332	4,264	10,188	880	92	*Private*
8	Atria Senior Living	14,249	11,168	2,358	1,223	124	*Private*
9	Capital Senior Living	10,780	3,834	6,946	589	77	**Public**
10	Assisted Living Concepts	9,305	-	-	-	211	**Public**
11	Senior Lifestyle Corp.	8,656	1,417	6,987	252	67	*Private*
12	Merrill Gardens	7,700	7,700	7,700	-	56	*Private*
13	One Eighty/Leisure Care	7,073	5,357	1,716	68	36	*Private*
14	Century Park Associates	6,143	2,497	3,646	-	48	*Private*
15	Brightview Senior Living	6,087	1,164	4,873	282	53	*Private*
16	Erickson Living	6,053	1,119	4,934	-	16	*Private*
17	VI Living	5,841	1,004	4,837	214	19	*Private*
18	USA Properties Fund	5,519	-	5,519	-	37	*Private*
19	Integral Senior Living	5,330	4,535	795	1,060	48	*Private*
20	Watermark Retirement	5,233	1,491	3,288	454	25	*Private*

Source: Largest Senior Living Providers by Anya Martin, May/June 2011 Assisted Living Executive.

Nursing Homes are a mature industry being subjected to competition from lower-cost alternatives.

Nursing Homes is a mature industry. There were an estimated 15,884 nursing homes, 67.5 percent for profit, in the United States in 2009 - 426 (2.6 percent) less than in 2005. Growth has been flat in all sizes of nursing homes. Demand for nursing home care and occupancies have decreased. Patients now have more options. Reimbursement for care in lower-cost alternative care settings has become more available. This is not a highly concentrated industry, the largest nursing home group, Golden Ventures, managed 325 nursing homes, 1.6 percent of total U.S. nursing homes. Highly integrated hospital systems, which increased their nursing home ownership 84.4 percent between 2001 and 2010, only controlled 817, about five percent, of U.S. nursing homes in 2010. Nursing homes are a local industry and competition is catchment area by catchment area specific. Consolidation has been in part hindered by CON (Certificate of Need) marketplace requirements in 36 states. Shared economies of scale exist with hospitals/hospital groups, etc.

Nursing Homes Lifecycle

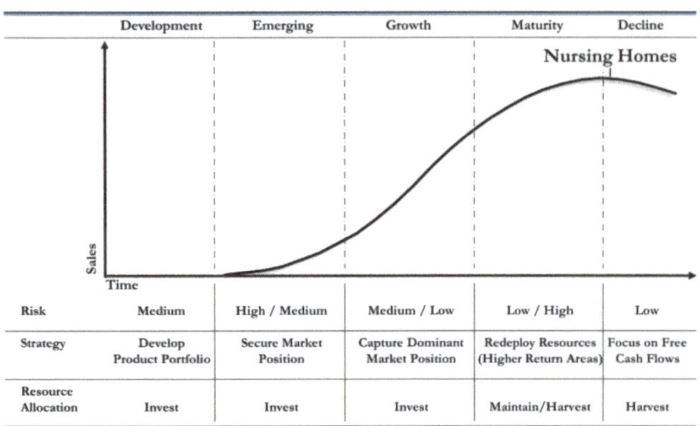

Source: MMC International

Nursing Homes By Bed Size

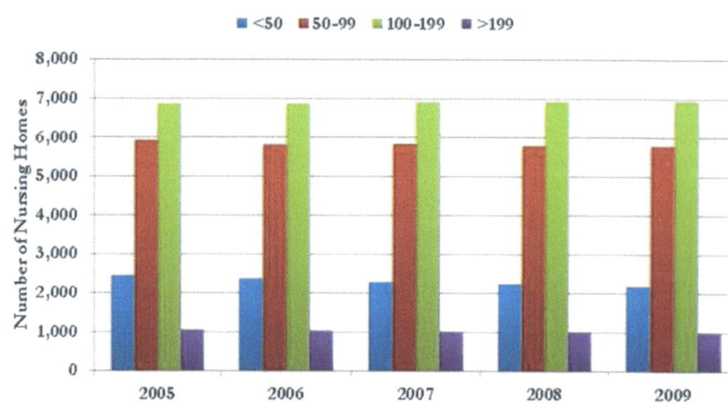

Source: MMC International and Nursing Home Data Compilation 2010 by CMS.

Number Of Nursing Homes

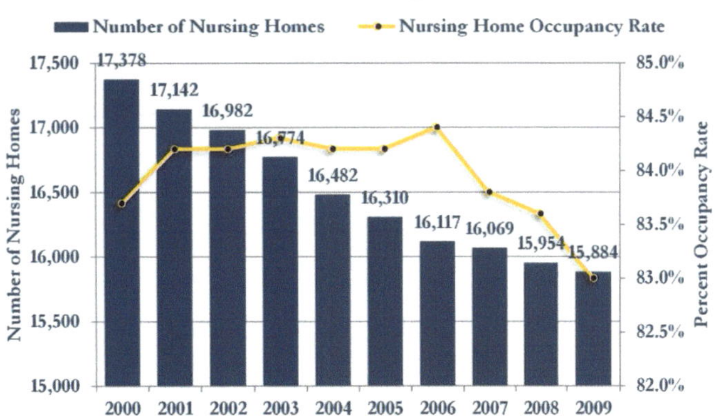

Source: MMC International and Nursing Home Data Compilation 2010 by CMS.

Nursing Homes By Ownership Type

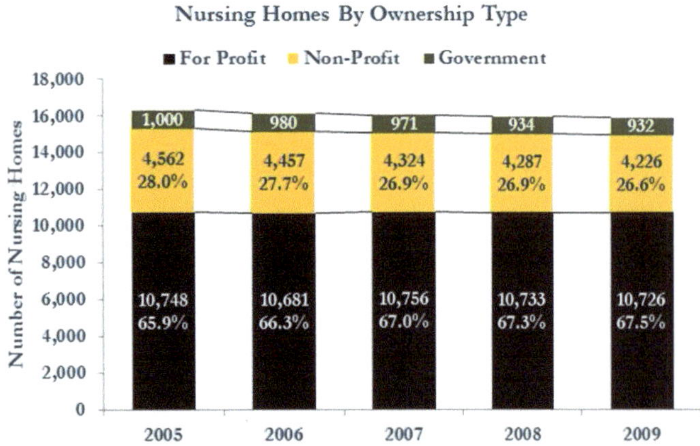

Source: MMC International and Nursing Home Data Compilation 2010 by CMS.

Rank	Group	Facilities	Percent of Total
1	Golden Ventures	325	1.6%
2	HCR Manor-Care Health Services	299	1.4%
3	Sunrise Senior Living	195	0.9%
4	Kindred Healthcare	213	1.0%
5	Life Care Centers of America	204	1.0%
6	Sun Health Care	196	0.9%
7	Evangelical Lutheran Good Sam	190	0.9%
8	Sava Senior Care	189	0.9%
9	Extendicare Health Services Inc	150	0.7%
10	Five Star Quality Care	146	0.7%
11	Brookdale Senior Living	110	0.5%
12	Fundamental	96	0.5%
13	National Healthcare Corp	81	0.4%
14	Emeritus Corp	78	0.4%
15	Life Care Services	73	0.3%
16	Americare	70	0.3%
17	Atria Senior Living Group	64	0.3%
18	Daybreak Venture	62	0.3%
19	Benchmark Assisted Living	46	0.2%
20	Coastal Administrative Services	45	0.2%
	Total Top 20 Groups	2,832	13.6%
	Total U.S. Nursing Homes	20,858	

Sources: MMC International and SK&A, A Cegedim Company, count data.

Home Healthcare is a growth industry being redefined by new technologies and an aging U.S. population.

Traditional home healthcare will be transformed by new telehealth and remote monitoring technologies between 2012 and 2020. The industry is in the growth phase of its lifecycle. Expansion is being driven by for-profit agencies which grew from 2,835 agencies in 2001, 41% of all agencies, to 6,585, 62% of all agencies in 2009. The new technologies will increasingly benefit from economies of scale in purchasing, maintenance, disease management, patient education, patient management, and administration. They will leverage nursing and medical staff, increasing productivity while decreasing overall costs per outcome per patient. This will open a round of consolidations of home health agencies between 2012 and 2020. No company owns more than seven percent of home healthcare agencies. How consolidation will transpire will be dependent upon reimbursement, how care is organized in each respective catchment area, and by CON regulations in the 17 states that have them. A home health care agency provides services that require a licensed professional - such as a registered nurse or physical, respiratory or occupational therapist - and a physician's prescription. These medical services are provided in the patient's home and can involve care for chronic health conditions or temporary care, as in the case of someone recovering from surgery or an injury. This is the least expensive care outside of self or family care.

Home Healthcare

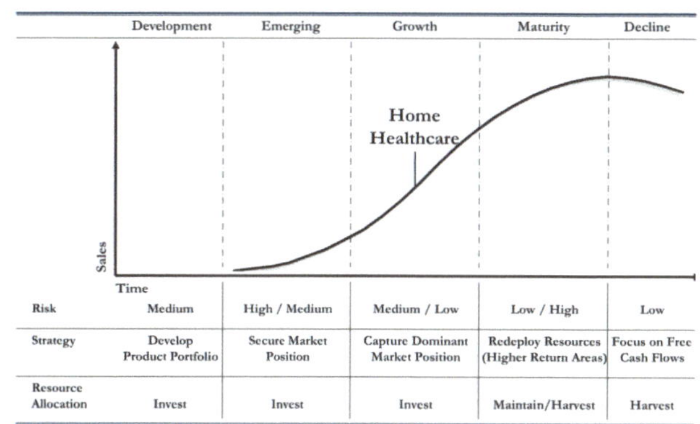

Source: MMC International.

Number of Medicare-Certified Home Care Agencies, By Auspice, 2000-2009

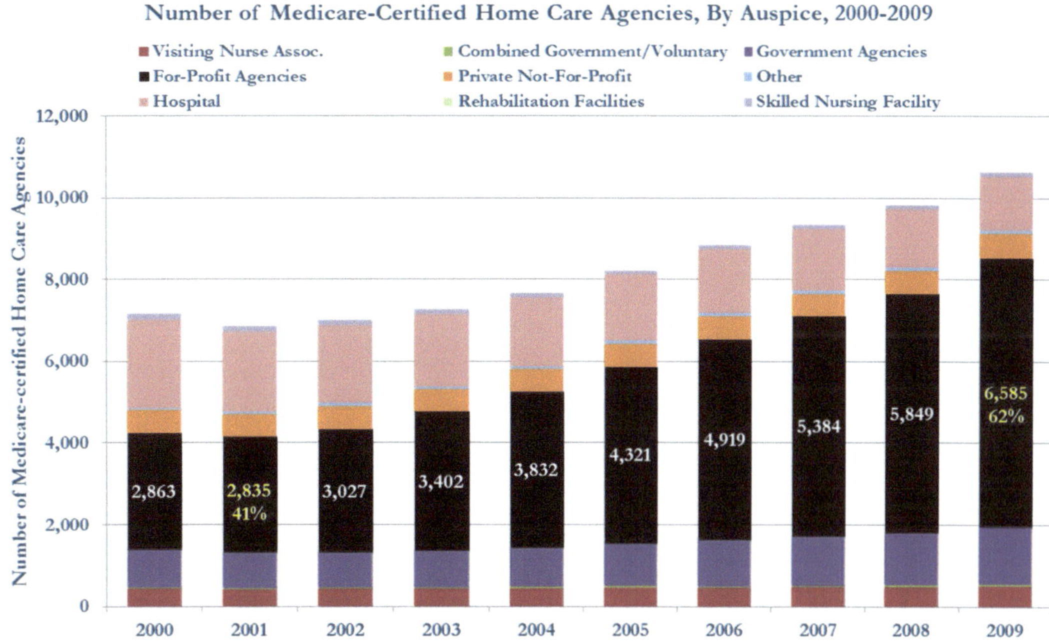

Sources: National Association for Home Care & Hospice and MMC International.

In 2010 there were 11,106 Medicare-certified home health agencies, which is the focus of this review, and 18,379 "assistance with daily-living" companies. The 18,739 agencies offer non-medical homecare, light housekeeping, companionship services, bathing, grooming, dressing, meal help, live in care, and care needs assessment, etc. The 11,106 Medicare-certified homes offer a wide range of skilled medical services such as skilled nursing care, physical therapy and occupational therapy from qualified medical professionals in addition to various services from home health aides. They may also include speech therapy, medical social workers, and specialized nursing programs, e.g. cardiac, diabetes, pain management, wound care, infusion therapy, oncology, and psychiatric services. They can also provide a portfolio of chronic care clinical programs designed from evidence-based best practices for patients with chronic diseases. Services may also include hospice, medical equipment, respiratory therapy, etc.

Federal and State governments pay for 80% of home healthcare expenditures.

The growing number of aging patients with their chronic conditions want to stay at home. They will drive demand for home care services. BB&T Capital Markets forecasted that the home healthcare industry will grow at nine percent annually through 2020. Medicare, Medicaid, and state and local governments pay for approximately 80 percent of United States home healthcare expenditures which totaled $72 billion in 2010. Private insurance covered eight percent. New technologies, laptop connectivity, point-of-care systems, and home telehealth provides agencies with the ability to reach more patients, reach them quicker, provide the clinician the tools needed for good practice, efficiency, and positive patient outcomes, and to conduct disease management. State Medicaid programs and commercial payers nationwide have recognized the benefits and are reimbursing for telehealth visits. Demonstration projects are occurring that assess the cost-effectiveness of home telehealth in Medicare and Veterans Administration patients. Without these advanced technologies, agencies will not be able to keep up with the steady influx of the aging baby boomers. The increased costs for the new devices and equipment have been shown to be more than offset by savings from decreases in physician visits and hospitalizations. Reimbursement will dictate the speed of technology adoption and the evolution of services and offerings by home healthcare agencies. Consolidation will be driven by competition.

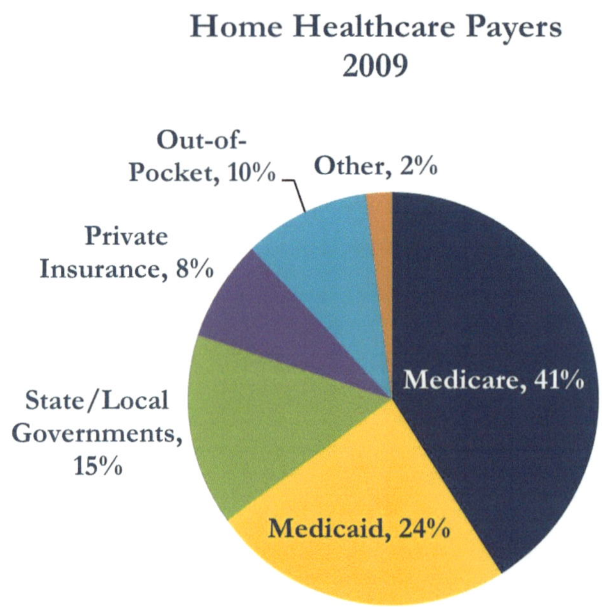

Source: Centers for Medicare & Medicaid Services, Office of the Actuary, National Healthcare Expenditures, www.cms.gov, March 2010 – 2009 is projected **data.**

Top 12 Home Healthcare Groups

Visiting Nurse Association
Apria Health Care
Interim Healthcare
Gentiva Health Services
Hospital Home Health Care
Option Care
Coram Healthcare
Amedisys
American HomePatient Care
Area Agency on Aging
Visiting Nurse Service
Lincare

17 INTERMEDIARIES

Intermediaries will be under increasing pressure to decrease costs - otherwise they will be circumvented.

Consolidation and innovation by payers, providers and manufacturers will increase downward price pressure on intermediaries such as pharmacy benefit management companies (PBMs), group purchasing organizations (GPOs), drug and medical products wholesalers, and drug stores. This will prompt the companies to innovate to retain or increase profitability, invest in diversification strategies to insure growth and sustainability, and programs to try to retain share. It will also push consolidation in unconsolidated sectors.

Over 96 percent of managed care plans use PBM services to help manage their drug benefits.

In 2009, over 96 percent of healthcare plans utilized various Pharmacy Benefit Management (PBM) services to manage their drug benefits. The 40 company 2011 PBM industry, which is approximately 52% of the way to industry maturity, will be in a period of increasing consolidation through 2020. Consolidation is expected to be driven by Express Scripts/Medco, CVS Caremark, UnitedHealth Group (OptumRx), Prime Therapeutics and the largest healthcare insurance companies. Shared economies of scale will play a significant role in the consolidation of the PBM market. Consolidating insurers, such as United Healthcare, have the ability to extract administrative and profit contributions paid for PBM services through vertical integration. As an example, United Healthcare intends to manage its 22.1 million Rx members through its OptumRX PBM when its contract with Medco expires in 2012 - positioning itself as a top ten PBM company at that time. If the merger between the largest and second largest PBMs, Express Scripts and Medco, is approved, the combined company will have revenues of $110 billion, manage prescription drug benefits for more the 115 million people, and handle one of every three prescriptions filled in the United States. The merged entity would also become the largest supplier of mail-order drugs to patients with chronic conditions and costly specialty drugs for conditions like H.I.V., hemophilia and rheumatoid arthritis. Express Scripts/Medco and CVS/Caremark have amassed sufficient critical mass to put historic PBM competitors at a cost disadvantage. PBMs, such as Prime Therapeutics which is collectively owned by 12 Blue Cross and Blue Shield plans with 17 million members, are in a position to further capture more business from Blue Cross and Blue Shield Plans. In turn, over the next ten years there will be fewer but more powerful PBMs for payers and pharmaceutical companies to deal with. Consolidation will facilitate manufacturers' efforts to forge creative agreements to benefit both the PBMs and their clients and the manufacturer.

U.S. PBM Industry Lifecycle

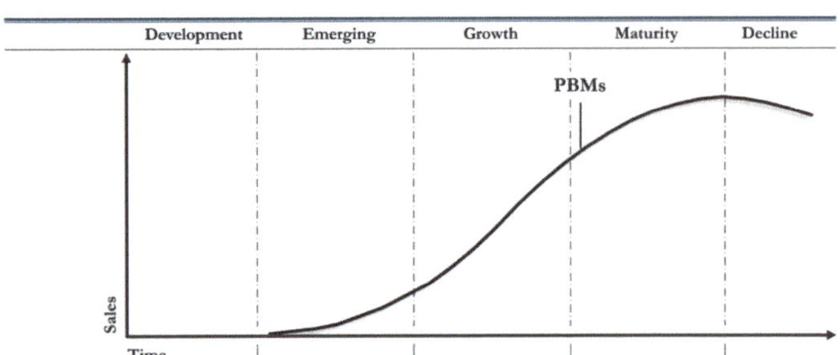

	Development	Emerging	Growth	Maturity	Decline
Risk	Medium	High / Medium	Medium / Low	Low / High	Low
Strategy	Develop Product Portfolio	Secure Market Position	Capture Dominant Market Position	Redeploy Resources (Higher Return Areas)	Focus on Free Cash Flows
Resource Allocation	Invest	Invest	Invest	Maintain/Harvest	Harvest

Source: MMC International.

U.S. 2010 PBM Covered Lives Relative Market Shares

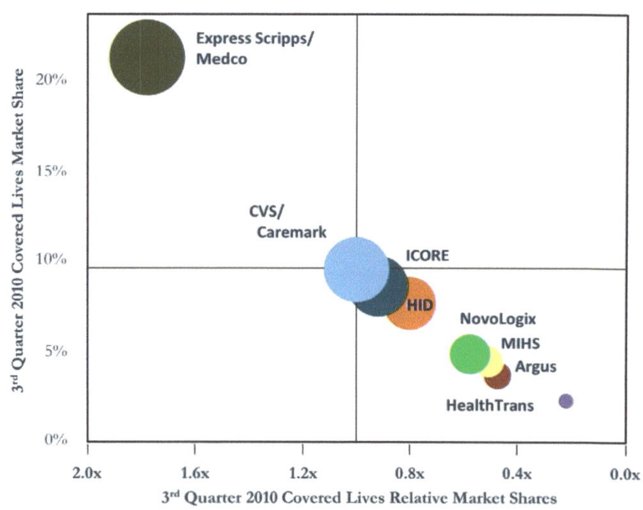

Source: MMC International.

Top 10 PBM Companies Represented 74.8% of PBM Covered Lives and 75.0% of Prescriptions as of the 3rd Quarter 2010

Company	Rx Covered Lives In Millions	% Market Share	Total Rx/ Year In Millions	% Market Share
Express Scripts, Inc./Medco*	155.0	23.2%	1,144.3	30.0%
CVS/Caremark Rx, Inc.	85.1	12.7%	658.5	17.3%
ICORE Healthcare, Inc.	60.0	9.0%	-	-
Health Information Designs, Inc.	52.0	7.8%	-	-
NovoLogix	40.0	6.0%	-	-
MedImpact Healthcare Systems, Inc.	32.0	4.8%	170.4	4.5%
Argus Health Systems, Inc.	28.6	4.3%	504.0	13.2%
Catalyst Rx (Walgreens Health Services)	16.2	2.4%	149.0	4.6%
HealthTrans	15.1	2.3%	90.1	2.4%
Prime Therapeutics LLC	15.0	2.3%	114.0	3.0%

Sources: Data from Atlantic Information Services' (AIS) exclusive quarterly survey of pharmacy benefit management companies conducted by Drug Benefit News during the 3rd quarter of 2010. HealthLeaders InterStudy, and analytics by MMC International.

Group purchasing organizations (GPOs) offerings and business practices are evolving with the market.

Group purchasing organizations (GPOs), a maturing industry, assist hospitals and healthcare providers in securing larger purchasing discounts and managing the supply chain for pharmaceuticals, durable medical and home equipment, medical and surgical supplies, laboratory supplies, physician preference products (e.g., orthopedic and cardiovascular devices), office supplies, nutritionals, and other ancillary products and contract services. GPOs consolidated into a handful of national groups in the 1980s and 1990s. The thinking was that the larger GPOs would have more contracting leverage with suppliers and as a result they would get better/lower prices. Two key components were missing: 1) the GPOs had no real leverage to get GPO members to purchase specified products in order to guarantee a certain volume in return for a better price - this was especially true for physician preference products, and 2) some products, e.g., medical gas, perishable food, equipment maintenance, and medical waste, etc., are best sourced on a regional basis. In the last few years, GPOs have gone from being simply a portfolio of prices to a service-oriented partner in the effort to drive expense out of the supply chain and other healthcare cost centers. The trend now is for the largest GPOs to offer value analysis, revenue cycle management, patient safety, IT systems, etc. to synergistically complement their purchasing activities. They are coordinating the supply chain with the clinical practice. They are also shopping for non-name brand suppliers with comparable products and devices to commoditize products/product groups to lower costs. To address local requirements (especially in rural versus metropolitan areas), improve local coordination, and to try to increase contract compliance in order to be able to get higher discounts for delivering higher volumes to manufacturers, the large national chains have enabled the formation of regional GPOs by strategically aligning with them and providing them with the benefits of their purchasing prowess. This, like Apple's opening up the iPhone and iPad to third-party apps, is forecast to result in more innovation by the regional and national GPOs and increased demand for the largest GPOs. Provider consolidations between 2012 and 2020 is expected to result in increased market shares and changed market positions for the largest GPOs - moving GPOs toward an oligopoly.

Top Nine Group Purchasing Organizations (GPOs)
Based Upon 2011 Average Purchased Volume

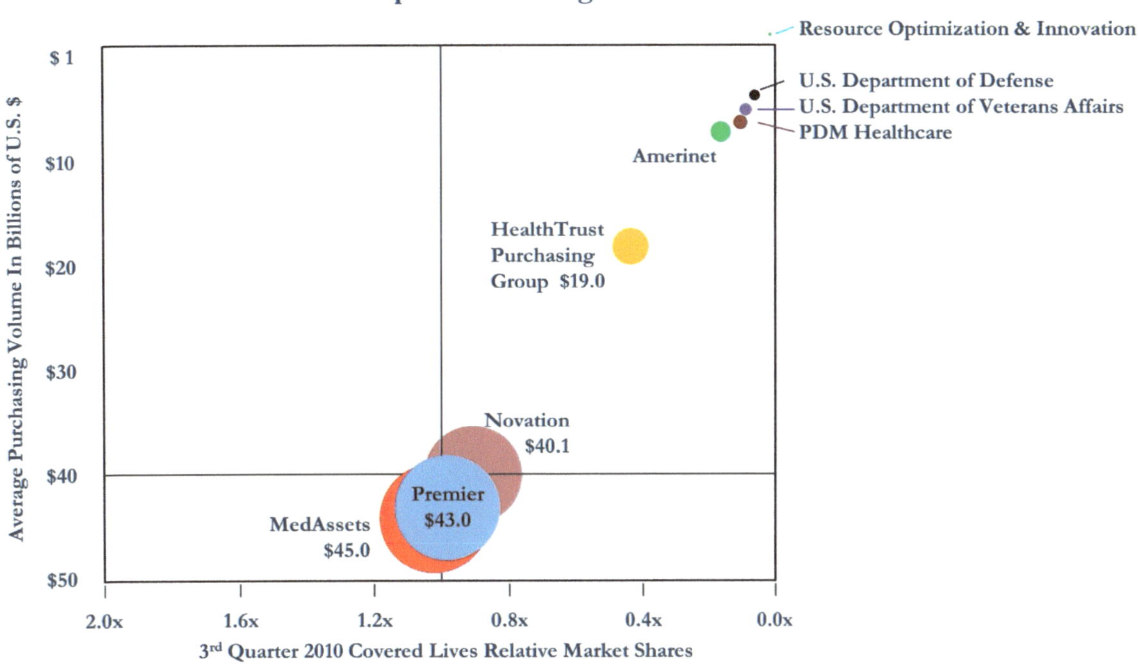

Note:

- Novation is owned by VHA Inc. and University HealthSystem Consortium. Its total includes contracted purchasing volume for supplies and services for VHA, UHC and Provista LLC.
- PDM Healthcare declined to disclose its annual purchasing volume, due to its proprietary nature, but assisted in ranking itself based on an unaudited analysis of the aggregate member facilities budgeted-for goods and services.
- The U.S. Departments of Veterans Affairs and Defense typically purchase products via the same programs and suppliers but their annual purchasing volumes are independently listed and separately ranked.

Sources: Prepared by MMC International based upon Healthcare Purchasing News research via GPO self-reported data, October 2011.

Healthcare products wholesaling in the United States is a consolidating market.

Healthcare wholesalers and distributors is a mature industry. Drug and/or medical supplies wholesalers and distributors deliver medicines, pharmaceutical supplies, care management products, medical devices and medical equipment to pharmacies, hospitals, surgery centers, physician offices, and other healthcare providers. In addition, most provide less expensive private label products at equal to or better than brand quality. Healthcare wholesalers also provide value-added services designed to reduce costs, enhance efficiency and improve purchasing, inventory, and financial management related to physical product management. The drug and medical/surgical supply distribution industry in the United States is highly competitive and characterized by intense pricing pressure. The industry is dominated by national wholesalers which compete with a shrinking number of regional and local distributors, as well as customer self-distribution models (e.g., mass merchandisers like Walmart and chain drugstores like Walgreens). Competitive factors include market pricing, total delivered product cost, product availability, the ability to fill and invoice orders accurately, delivery time, range of services provided, efficient product sourcing, inventory management, information technology, electronic commerce capabilities, and the ability to meet special customer requirements. The leading companies, McKesson, Cardinal Health, AmerisourceBergen, Henry Schein, and Owens and Minor are all generating attractive free cash flows.

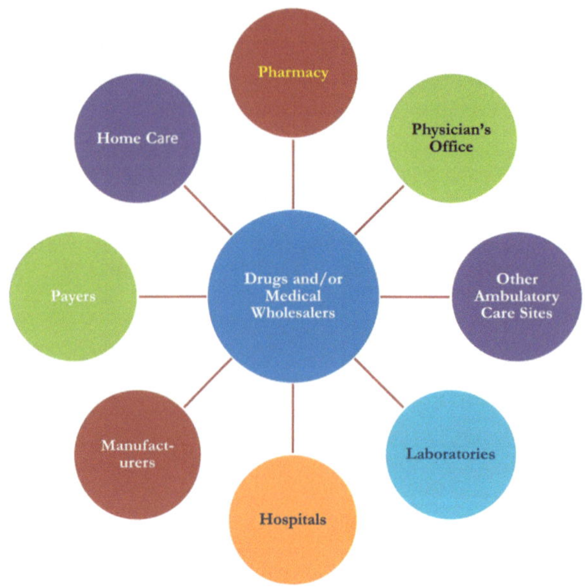

United States drug wholesaling is a mature $320 billion healthcare wholesale industry segment.

Drug wholesalers is a mature industry. Each major drug wholesaler has invested in additional product offerings to sustain their growth and profitability. These offerings afford each of the major drug wholesalers shared economies of scale. In turn, the shared economies are allowing three profitable dominant companies (McKesson Corporation with a 38.1 percent market share, Cardinal Health, Inc. with 33 percent, and AmerisourceBergen Corporation with 28.8 percent) in what is a mature industry. The three represented 85 percent, $272.4 billion, of United States pharmaceutical wholesaler revenues in 2010. Ongoing consolidation will mean fewer but larger pharmaceutical customers. Larger customers represent lower profit margins on brand-name drugs and customers that may bypass the drug wholesalers for certain services. Discount generic programs are shifting retail market share away from wholesaler-supplied dispensing channels into self-warehousing retailers, negatively impacting drug wholesaler profitability. Government agencies are also questioning the profits that the distribution channel earns from generic injectable drugs. Some pharmacy benefit managers (PBMs) are developing services that shift responsibility for specialty drug management from the medical benefit to the pharmacy benefit. Examples include Express Scripts and Medco Health Solutions. If successful, these programs will reduce the importance of specialty distribution channels by reducing the role of wholesalers in the purchase decision. Mergers of brand-name pharmaceutical manufacturers could reduce wholesaler payments under fee-for-service agreements. The consolidation of manufacturers is generally negative for wholesalers because a larger drug maker would have additional leverage in a fee-for-service negotiation. However, major branded drug patent expirations will favorably impact wholesaler margins between 2012 and 2020.

U.S. Drug Wholesalers Lifecycle

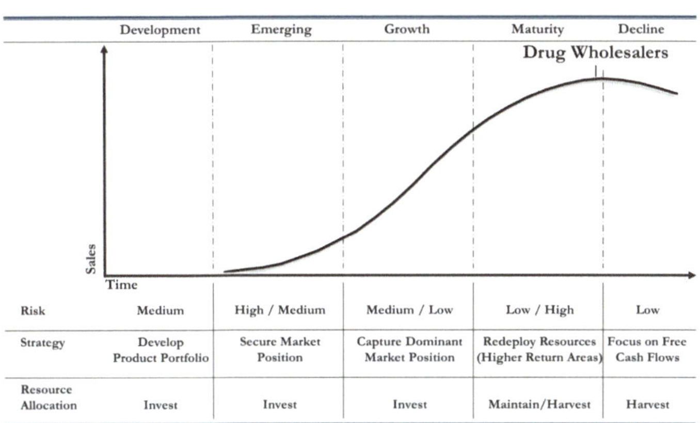

Source: MMC International.

U.S. Drug Wholesalers Concentration

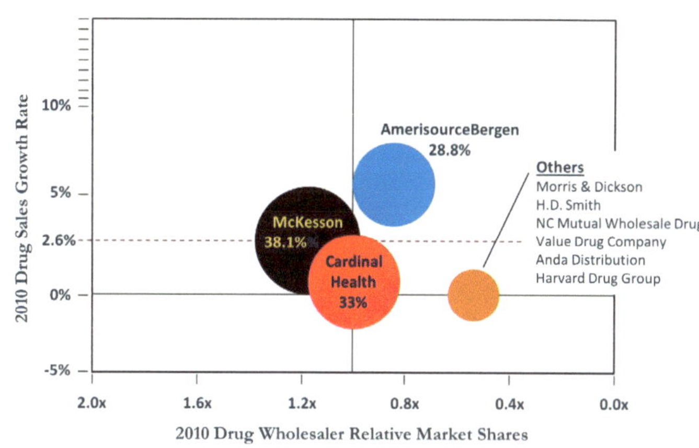

Source: MMC International.

All three of the major wholesalers:

- distribute branded and generic pharmaceutical, over-the-counter healthcare, and consumer products through its pharmaceutical distribution business to retailers (including chain and independent drug stores and pharmacy departments of supermarkets and mass merchandisers), hospitals, and alternate care providers (including mail order pharmacies).
- maintain prime vendor relationships that streamline the purchasing process resulting in greater efficiency and lower costs for customers.
- help pharmaceutical manufacturers with services including distribution, inventory management, data/reporting, new product launch support, and contract and chargeback administration.
- distribute specialty pharmaceutical products and provide services to pharmaceutical manufacturers, third-party payers and healthcare service providers supporting the marketing, distribution, and payment for specialty pharmaceutical products.
- franchise retail pharmacies (to provide economies of scale to independent pharmacies).
- provide pharmacy services to hospitals and other healthcare facilities.

The medical products wholesale operations benefit from shared scale economies with drug wholesaling.

The Medical segment distributes a broad range of medical, surgical and laboratory products to hospitals, surgery centers, laboratories, physician offices, nursing homes, home healthcare, extended care, occupational health facilities, other healthcare providers, and consumers (Owens and Minor is focusing on consumers). The dominant medical products wholesalers, McKesson, Cardinal, Owens and Minor, and Henry Schein also source and develop their own line of private brand medical and surgical products. Examples of manufactured products include: single-use surgical drapes, gowns and apparel; exam and surgical gloves, sterile and non-sterile procedure kits, fluid suction and collection systems, respiratory products (e.g., ventilation equipment and supplies), reusable surgical instruments and biopsy devices, patient identification systems, etc. In addition, the segment provides supply chain services, including spend management, distribution management, and inventory management services to healthcare providers. The industry leaders are in the process of segmenting the market, positioning themselves, or reinforcing their positions in the respective sectors where they are especially strong and/or where they can increase profitability and strengthen their marketplace positions. This is an indication of a maturing market where competitors try to carve out the most profitable market segments for themselves. Their investments then induce competitors to invest in those market segments which the market leader finds less attractive/a lower priority. Economies of scale will be playing an increasingly more important role as providers become bigger and purchasing becomes more consolidated – into integrated healthcare delivery systems and fewer and larger group purchasing organizations (GPOs).

Retail Pharmacies is a maturing industry which will be redefined between 2012 and 2020.

There were four billion prescriptions, representing $307.4 billion (at manufacturers' prices) dispensed in the United States in 2010, up 2.4 percent from $300.3 billion in 2009. The prescriptions were dispensed by >60,393 pharmacies (2009 count), excluding the PBM and health insurance company owned mail order pharmacies (hereinafter pharmacies). All pharmacies, including independent pharmacies, enjoy economies of scale in purchasing and distribution. Independents get their scale benefits via agreements with drug wholesalers and/or their independent pharmacy franchises, e.g., Cardinal Health's Medicine Shoppe® and Medicap® franchises and McKesson's Health Mart®. The advent of low-cost generics and looming patent expirations has shifted market competition and enabled Mass Merchandiser to use discounted or free generic prescriptions as promotional items to lure customers into their stores. The implications are most serious for Independent Drug Stores and Chain Drug Stores that depend on prescriptions for approximately 82.5 percent and 66.9 percent of total sales, respectively.

U.S. Prescription Market By Channel of Distribution

	In Billions of U.S. Dollars						Percent of U.S. Prescription Market By Channel					
	2006	2007	2008	2009	2010	2006-2010 % Growth	2006	2007	2008	2009	2010	2006-2010 Trend
Chain Drug Stores	91.9	96	99.7	105.4	108.1	17.6%	34.0%	34.2%	34.9%	35.1%	35.2%	
Mail Service Pharmacies	42.7	44.1	46.5	51.5	52.6	23.2%	15.8%	15.7%	16.3%	17.1%	17.1%	
Independent Drug Stores	36.5	37.5	36.9	37.3	37.9	3.8%	13.5%	13.4%	12.9%	12.4%	12.3%	
Clinics	29.8	32.7	33.0	34.8	36.2	21.5%	11.0%	11.7%	11.6%	11.6%	11.8%	
Non-Federal Hospitals	26.1	26.4	26.8	27.6	28.0	7.3%	9.7%	9.4%	9.4%	9.2%	9.1%	
Food Stores	21.9	21.5	20.4	21.2	21.3	-2.7%	8.1%	7.7%	7.1%	7.1%	6.9%	
Long-Term Care	12.8	13.3	13.7	13.8	14.8	15.6%	4.7%	4.7%	4.8%	4.6%	4.8%	
Federal Facilities	3.7	4	3.9	4.1	3.9	5.4%	1.4%	1.4%	1.4%	1.4%	1.3%	
Home Health Care	2.4	2.5	2.5	2.5	2.5	4.2%	0.9%	0.9%	0.9%	0.8%	0.8%	
HMO	1.6	1.5	1.3	1.1	1.1	-31.3%	0.6%	0.5%	0.5%	0.4%	0.4%	
Miscellaneous	0.9	1	1.0	1.0	1.0	11.1%	0.3%	0.4%	0.4%	0.3%	0.3%	
	270.3	280.5	285.7	300.3	307.4	13.7%	100.0%	100.0%	100.0%	100.0%	100.0%	

Source: IMS National Sales Perspectives™, April 7, 2011. Report reflects Prescription-bound products including Insulins (and excludes other products such as OTC).

Sales and Prescription Brands and Generics Market Shares

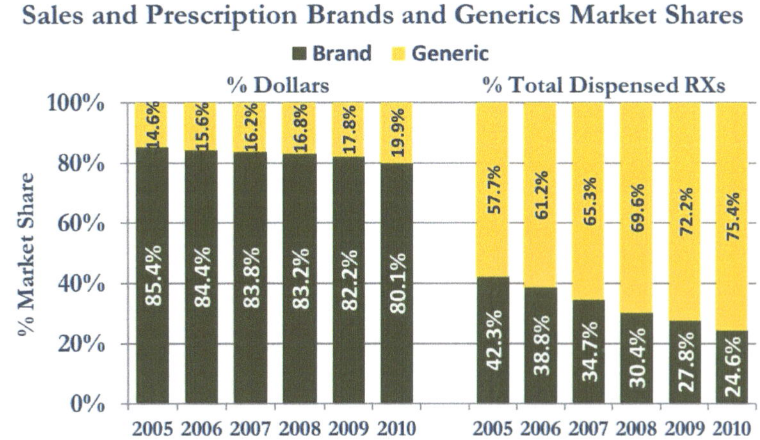

Sources: IMS National Sales Perspectives and National Prescription Audit.

Estimated Sales By Major Product Groups

	Prescription Drugs	OTC Products	Food	Health and Beauty Aids	General Merchandise
Chain Drug Stores	66.9%	7.0%	6.8%	6.0%	13.3%
Independent Drug Stores	82.5%	1.4%		0.6%	15.5%
Mass Merchandisers	6.3%	2.1%	16.8%	4.1%	70.7%
Supermarkets	13.6%	2.0%	71.5%	2.4%	10.5%

Sources: AC Nielsen, U.S. Department of Commerce Bureau of Economic Analysis and MMC International.

The consolidated Chain Drug retailer segment is the best positioned to increase its prescriptions share.

Chain Drug Stores, with a 35 percent 2010 prescription sales ($108.1 billion) market share and 37 percent of total pharmacies, is dominated by thee chains, Walgreens, CVS Caremark, and Rite Aid. The top three together represented 86 percent of total United States Chain Drug Store pharmacies in 2009. The three are positioned to continue to grow their respective industry market shares through new store openings, acquisition of independent pharmacies, and addition of preventive care services. The strong competition, driven by discounting programs by Mass Merchandisers like Wal-Mart will put significant pressure on independent pharmacies. This is expected to result in a decrease in the total number of independent pharmacies between 2012 and 2020. The Mass Merchandiser stores segment growth is relatively saturated. Growth will be in great part limited by the addition of new stores. Wal-Mart represents fifty-seven percent of Mass Merchandiser sales and forty-five percent of Mass Merchandiser pharmacies. Wal-Mart's pharmacy growth will be limited by new store openings as Wal-Mart has pharmacies in virtually all of its stores. The same goes for Target, the number two United States retailer, etc. Supermarkets are in the same position as Mass Merchandisers.

2009 Top 25 United States Pharmacy Chains Ranked By Number of Pharmacies

Rank	Companies	Chain		Independents		Mass Merchandiser		Supermarkets		Total	
		Stores	Share	Stores	Share	Stores	Share	Stores	Share	Stores	Share
1	Walgreens	7,420	33%							7,420	12%
2	CVS Caremark	7,074	32%							7,074	12%
3	Rite Aid	4,780	21%							4,780	8%
4	Wal-Mart					3,686	45%			3,686	6%
5	The Kroger Co.							1,960	21%	1,960	3%
6	Target Corporation					1,681	21%			1,681	3%
7	Safeway							1,330	14%	1,330	2%
8	Medicine Shoppe			1,225	6%					1,225	2%
9	Sears holding					1,025	13%			1,025	2%
10	Supervalu							860	9%	860	1%
11	Publix Super Markets							795	9%	795	1%
12	Ahold USA							668	7%	668	1%
13	Sam's Club					606	7%			606	1%
14	Costco Wholesale					466	6%			466	1%
15	Winn-Dixie Stores							403	4%	403	1%
16	Hy-Vee Inc.							222	2%	222	0%
17	Giant Eagle							207	2%	207	0%
18	Great Atlantic & Pacific Tea Co.							204	2%	204	0%
19	Meijer					190	2%			190	0%
20	H.E. Butt Grocery Co.							188	2%	188	0%
21	Albertson LLC							156	2%	156	0%
22	Save Mart Supermarkets							156	2%	156	0%
23	USA Drug	144	1%							144	0%
24	Pamida Stores					142	2%			142	0%
25	ShopKo Stores					140	2%			140	0%
	Sub-Total	19,418	87%	1,225	6%	7,936	98%	7,149	78%	35,728	59%
	Others	2,849	13%	19,567	94%	201	2%	2,048	22%	24,665	41%
	Total	22,267	100%	20,792	100%	8,137	100%	9,197	100%	60,393	100%

Sources: AC Nielsen, U.S. Department of Commerce Bureau of Economic Analysis, NACDS Economics Department, and MMC International.

18 PHARMACEUTICALS

Pharmaceuticals are an opportunity-rich industry which will be fundamentally transformed by 2020.

The United States represented thirty-six percent, $307 billion, of the $856 billion worldwide pharmaceutical market in 2010. In 2011, there were over 3,000 pharmaceutical, biotechnology, and generics companies, universities, colleges, and hospitals involved in the development of about 2,900 compounds to potentially treat 9,171 diseases or conditions in development in the United States. Four hundred eighty-eight companies of the 3,000 entities sold more than 6,100 different FDA (Food and Drug Administration) approved prescription and OTC (over-the-counter) drugs. The industry is comprised of a myriad of technology, therapy, product, customer, and market segments. Products can be segmented by branded (innovative/protected products), generic and, OTC drugs. The business is global; however, marketing success requires adaptation to local regulatory and market requirements. Innovative pharmaceuticals, which is comprised of traditional small molecule proteins and biotechnology drugs, is at the beginning of the transition from selling products to selling patient outcomes – to personalized medicine. It is transitioning from a historic focus on small molecule chemicals to biotechnology-driven personalized medicine. Existing medicines in 2011addressed only some 207 different targets, whereas there are more than two million proteins in the human body which may potentially cause diseases. The migration to personalized medicine and biotechnology is being enabled by the convergence of: 1) genomics, 2) systems biology (disease pathways), 3) diagnostics and biomarkers, 4) improving drug delivery systems, 5) electronic health records and national health information exchanges, 6) dynamic and more powerful data mining, 7) increasingly fewer but larger payers/customers, 8) a movement towards reimbursement for outcomes, and 9) efforts by the U.S. Food and Drug Administration (FDA) to streamline regulatory processes over the next few years to come more in line with changing pharmaceutical R&D. Generics, which is an economies of scale, cost- and price-driven business, is made up of different product types and customer groups. Customer choice is based upon quality, the breadth of the product line, and cost. All segments of the U.S. pharmaceutical industry, branded pharmaceuticals, biotechnology, and generics, will be fundamentally restructured over the next ten years. For many innovative companies, with product portfolios that will lose patent protection for a large number of products, the rules related to a maturing industry will come into play. This will continue until a new industry redefines what had been the traditional pharmaceutical, biotechnology and generics industries. Success will require new strategies, competencies and organizational structures. The key to success in pharmaceuticals is properly defining the market in which the company competes and the core competencies that the company has and will require. The $856 billion 2010 global pharmaceutical market, which will be entering a period of reemergence between 2012 and 2020, will increasingly be opportunity rich. However, the rules and requirements for success will be irreversibly changed between 2012 and 2020.

U.S. pharmaceuticals are a maturing industry that will be revitalized between 2012 and 2020.

The overall U.S. pharmaceutical industry entered the mature phase of its industry lifecycle in 2002 – future U.S. growth will come from pipeline products, improving patient prescription persistence and compliance, repurposing of existing drugs or drugs that failed clinical trials – all enabled by improved sub-population data analysis and the emerging "pharmaceutical care" industry. Personalized medicine will allow the pharmaceutical companies to begin shifting from selling drugs to marketing cost-effective outcomes. Outcomes based marketing, while more complex, will allow drug compensation based upon efficacy. This opens up the opportunity for pharmaceutical companies to share in the cost savings to the healthcare system evidenced by proper drug prescribing, and patient prescription persistence and compliance.

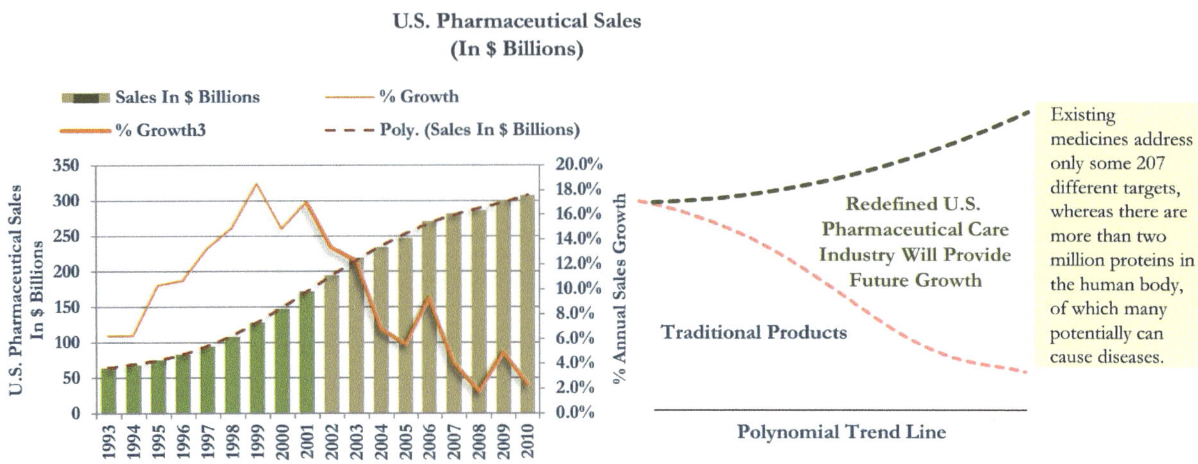

Sources: MMC International and IMS Health annual sales statistics 1993 to 2010.

- The maturing of the U.S. pharmaceutical market, the largest pharmaceuticals country market worldwide (36% of global sales in 2010), signals accelerated worldwide industry consolidation between 2012 and 2020.
  - Mergers and acquisitions activity will be focused on acquiring products, technologies and local country market presence – mainly on smaller transactions, not on mega-mergers.
- Growth outside of the United States will result in downward pressures and increased scrutiny regarding U.S. market investments/resource allocations.
- The "Pharmerging" tier one and two country markets (China, Brazil, India and Russia), generics and specialty markets represent growth opportunities for the traditional U.S. pharmaceutical industry over the next ten years.
  - The tier three markets (Venezuela, Poland, Argentina, Turkey, Mexico, Vietnam, South Africa, Thailand, Indonesia, Romania, Egypt, Pakistan and Ukraine), each with ≥$1.5 billion in annual incremental brand sales, also represent growth opportunities.

Small molecule chemicals are being replaced by biotechnology-based therapies.

Small molecule chemicals appear to have reached their technology productivity returns limit. They are rapidly being replaced by biotechnology-based therapies. Traditional pharmaceutical and biotechnology companies will merge over the next ten years to create an integrated industry. Biotech drugs (therapeutic protein hormones, cytokines, tissue growth factors, monoclonal antibodies, cell or gene therapies, and vaccines) will soon dominate the pharmaceutical industry. Financial community analyst projections indicate that eight of the top ten selling therapies in 2014 will be products of genetic engineering - while only two are traditional oral pills made through chemical synthesis.

NME versus Biologics Approvals
1999 to 2010

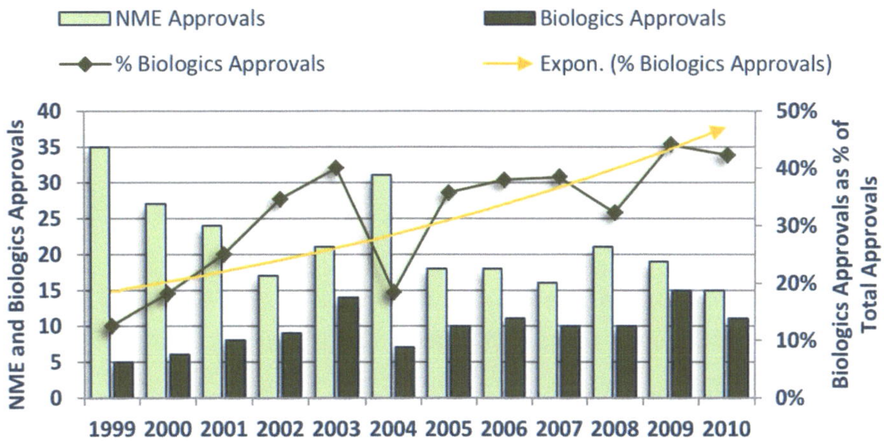

Sources: Food and Drug Administration (FDA), FDA Center for Drugs Evaluation and Research (CDER), Center for Biologics Evaluation and Research (CBER), Evaluate Pharma, and MMC International Analytics.

The decreasing 1999 to 2010 new drug approvals trend is indicative of a maturing industry.

The pharmaceutical industry is in the transition from separate pharmaceutical, biotechnology and generics industries into a redefined integrated pharmaceutical care industry - which will be defined by personalized medicine. Large pharmaceutical companies have the financial resources to invest in and acquire biotechnology companies to revitalize their companies. Simultaneously, biotechnology companies need the financial, regulatory, R&D, manufacturing, distribution, and marketing and sales resources that traditional pharmaceutical companies can provide. The large generic companies have the cash flows and stock valuations to diversify their offerings to include innovative products. The direction is clearly towards more licensing and merger activity between 2012 and 2020 as pharmaceutical companies innovate to retain or improve their respective market positions. However, strategic alliances, licensing and mergers and acquisitions between existing companies is insufficient to revitalize the industry. Changes in how R&D is conducted and how products are approved will be the keys to the creation of a revitalized industry.

An inability to replace high revenue and profitability products, from internal research and/or in-licensing, due to the decreasing R&D productivity trend, depresses company valuations and makes them attractive acquisitions. Acquisitions also become an avenue for filling pipeline/sales shortfalls.

Total New Medical Entities (NMEs) and Biologics (BLA) Approvals Versus Five Year Estimated Peak Sales

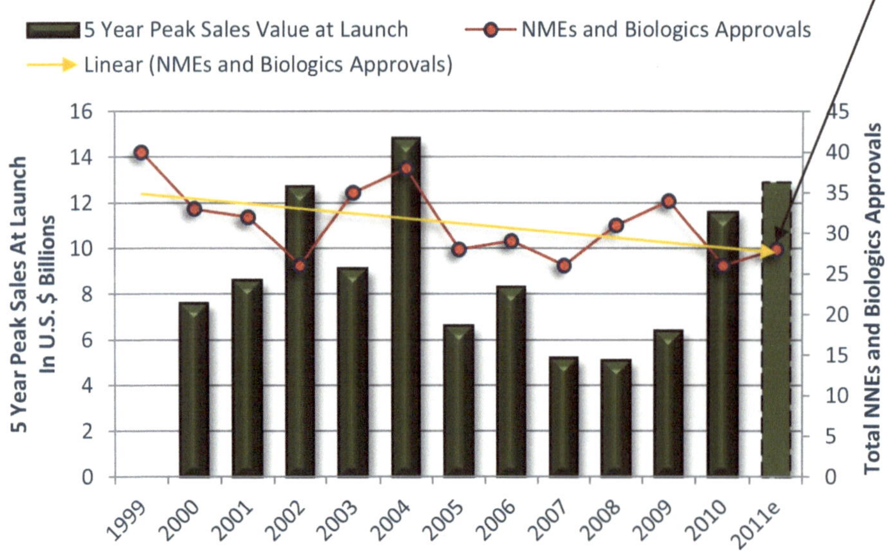

Sources: Food and Drug Administration (FDA), FDA Center for Drugs Evaluation and Research (CDER), Center for Biologics Evaluation and Research (CBER), Evaluate Pharma, and MMC International Analytics.

The importance of the Center for Biologics Evaluation and Research (CBER) will continue to increase.

Average first-in-class therapeutic competition now materializes two years after initial market entry.

Another indicator of a maturing pharmaceutical industry is the level of competition. By 1995, nearly all the new "first-in-class" pharmaceuticals faced a competitive product in at least Phase II testing at product launch. By 2009, the average time for a first-in-class drug to encounter competition had been decreased to two years. This in part explains why the majority of new products fail to earn a risk-adjusted return on the investments made to develop them. Simultaneously, the growth and consolidation of generics companies has resulted in more brand patents being challenged. However, the average period of protection before generic competition materializes has remained at 11.5 years.

Illustrative Pharmaceutical Lifecycle
New pharmaceutical medicines face competition after a relatively short period on the market.

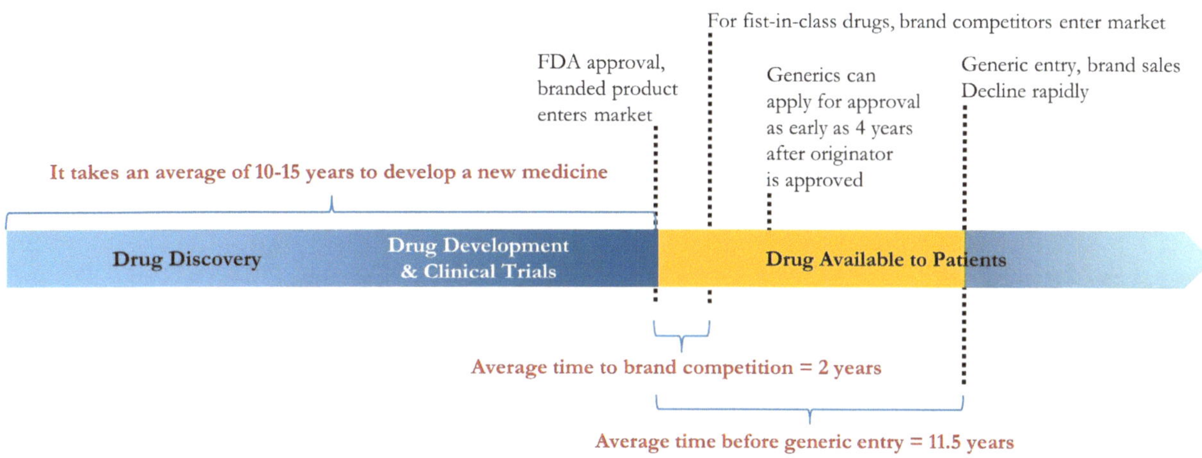

Source: Pharmaceutical Research and Manufacturers of America analysis (2009).

Most <u>major</u> drug classes were adequately served by generics in 2011, virtually all will be by 2015.

Virtually all major drug classes, except respiratory and cancer agents, will be adequately served by generics by 2015. Most major drug classes were adequately served by generics in 2011. Existing medicines address only some 207 different targets, whereas there are more than two million proteins in the human body. Many potentially can cause diseases. These factors explain why pharmaceutical research has shifted its focus to specialty pharmaceuticals, especially cancer agents, over the last few years. According to IMS Health, specialty drugs will account for 40 percent of national drug spending by 2014. The market shift to specialty drugs is the reason many industry observers feel that the strategy to focus on blockbuster drugs, those with greater than one billion dollars in potential global peak annual sales, is no longer viable. However, the shift to personalized medicine, selling outcomes versus drugs, is expected to result in the introduction of niche products with companion biomarkers that will generate over one billion dollars in annual global sales. The trend to a redefined industry will be accelerated by major patent expirations between 2012 and 2020. The patents on the 20 largest selling products worldwide will all have expired by 2017.

■ = Drug Class   = Generic Products   ■ = Brand Declining Prescriptions   ■ = Brand w/Increasing Prescriptions   **Bold Text** = Branded Product

DRUG CLASS/PRODUCT	Brand/ Generic	Patent Expiration	Total Prescriptions In Millions 2008	2009	2010	08 To 10 Trend
ANTIDEPRESSANTS						
Sertraline	Generic		22.0	22.2	23.0	
Lexapro	**Brand**	**2012**	21.1	19.4	17.5	
Citalopram Hydrobromide	Generic		13.6	16.3	17.4	
Fluoxetine	Generic		16.3	15.8	15.8	
Trazadone	Generic				11.2	
ANTIHYPERTENSIVES						
Lisinopril	Generic		45.1	46.7	46.9	
Amlodipine Besylate	Generic		23.7	27.2	29.4	
Hydrochlorothiazide	Generic		31.0	30.0	28.5	
Atenolol	Generic		28.1	25.1	21.7	
Metoprolol Succinate ER	Generic		24.8	23.3	20.7	
ANTI-INFECTIVES						
Mupirocin	Generic		2.9	3.3	3.5	
Clindamycin Topical	Generic		1.9	2.1	2.2	
Metronidazole Vaginal	Generic		0.6	0.7	0.9	
Bactroban	**Brand**	**2014**	1.1	0.8	0.7	
Metronidazole Topical	Generic		0.7	0.7	0.7	
ANTIPSYCHOTICS						
Seroquel	**Brand**	**2012**	6.5	6.2	5.6	
Risperidone	Generic		0.0	3.4	3.8	
Abilify	**Brand**	**2015**	2.6	3.3	3.7	
Zyprexa	**Brand**	**2011**	2.0	1.8	1.6	
Geodon Oral	**Brand**	**2012**	1.2	1.2	1.1	
BENIGN PROSTATIC HYPERPLASIA						
Flomax	**Brand**		8.4	8.0	5.7	
Finasteride	Generic		2.4	2.6	2.8	
Doxazosin	Generic		3.5	3.3	2.8	
Terazosin	Generic		2.7	2.5	2.7	
Avodart	**Brand**	**2015**	2.3	2.4	2.4	
CHEMOTHERAPEUTIC AGENTS						
Methotrexate	Generic		3.4	3.5	3.4	
Tretinoin	Generic		0.0	0.0	1.2	
Arimidex	**Brand**	**2012**	1.3	1.3	1.2	
Tamoxifen	Generic		1.2	1.2	1.2	
Femara	**Brand**	**2011**	0.8	0.8	0.8	

DRUG CLASS/PRODUCT	Brand/ Generic	Patent Expiration	Total Prescriptions In Millions 2008	2009	2010	08 To 10 Trend
CHOLESTEROL REDUCERS						
Simvastatin	Generic		36.9	46.8	50.1	
Lipitor	**Brand**	**2011**	39.9	34.2	28.3	
Crestor	**Brand**	**2016**	11.1	12.8	14.7	
Pravastatin	Generic		7.9	10.1	11.9	
Lovastatin	Generic		10.2	9.5	9.4	
GASTROINTESTINAL AGENTS						
Metoclopramide	Generic		4.1	3.9	3.0	
Dicyclomine Hydrochloride	Generic		2.1	2.4	2.4	
Asacol	**Brand**	**2021**	1.4	1.3	1.1	
Chlordiazepoxide with Clidinium	Generic		0.8	0.9	0.8	
Sulfasalazine	Generic		0.6	0.6	0.6	
GLAUCOMA						
Xalatan	**Brand**	**2011**	4.6	4.0	3.6	
Lumigan	**Brand**	**2014**	1.6	1.6	1.6	
Travatan Z	**Brand**	**2014**	0.6	1.0	1.2	
Dorzolamide Hydrocloride/Timolol Maleate	Generic				1.1	
Alphagan P	**Brand**	**2022**	1.6	1.4	1.0	
NONSTEROIDAL ANTI-INFLAMMATORY DRUGS						
Ibuprofen	Generic		18.0	17.8	17.1	
Meloxicam	Generic		7.5	9.0	9.2	
Naproxen	Generic		9.4	9.0	9.0	
Celebrex	**Brand**	**2014**	8.3	7.6	6.5	
Diclofenac Sodium SR	Generic		4.2	4.3	4.2	
RESPIRATORY AGENTS						
Singulair	**Brand**	**2012**	20.5	18.6	17.8	
ProAir HFA	**Brand**	**2023**	9.2	14.0	15.0	
Advair Diskus	**Brand**	**2016**	13.4	12.6	11.8	
Ventolin HFA	**Brand**	**2025**			6.7	
Albuterol Nebulizer Solution	Generic		5.4	5.5	6.0	
SYSTEMIC ANTIBIOTICS						
Azithromycin	Generic		38.3	37.5	37.2	
Amoxicillin	Generic		38.1	35.9	32.7	
Amoxicillin/Potassium Clavulanate	Generic		16.0	15.8	16.1	
Cephalexin	Generic		15.9	15.2	13.6	
Trimethoprim/Sulfamethoxazole	Generic				13.6	

Sources: MMC International, FDA Orange Book, and SDI data.

Patent expirations are good news for generics but not for branded and biotechnology companies.

The drugs that lost or will lose patent protection between 2010 and 2020 had sales of $149 billion in 2010. They represented 60% of the $249 billion 2010 branded U.S. pharmaceutical market. This is good news for generics but not for branded and biotech companies.

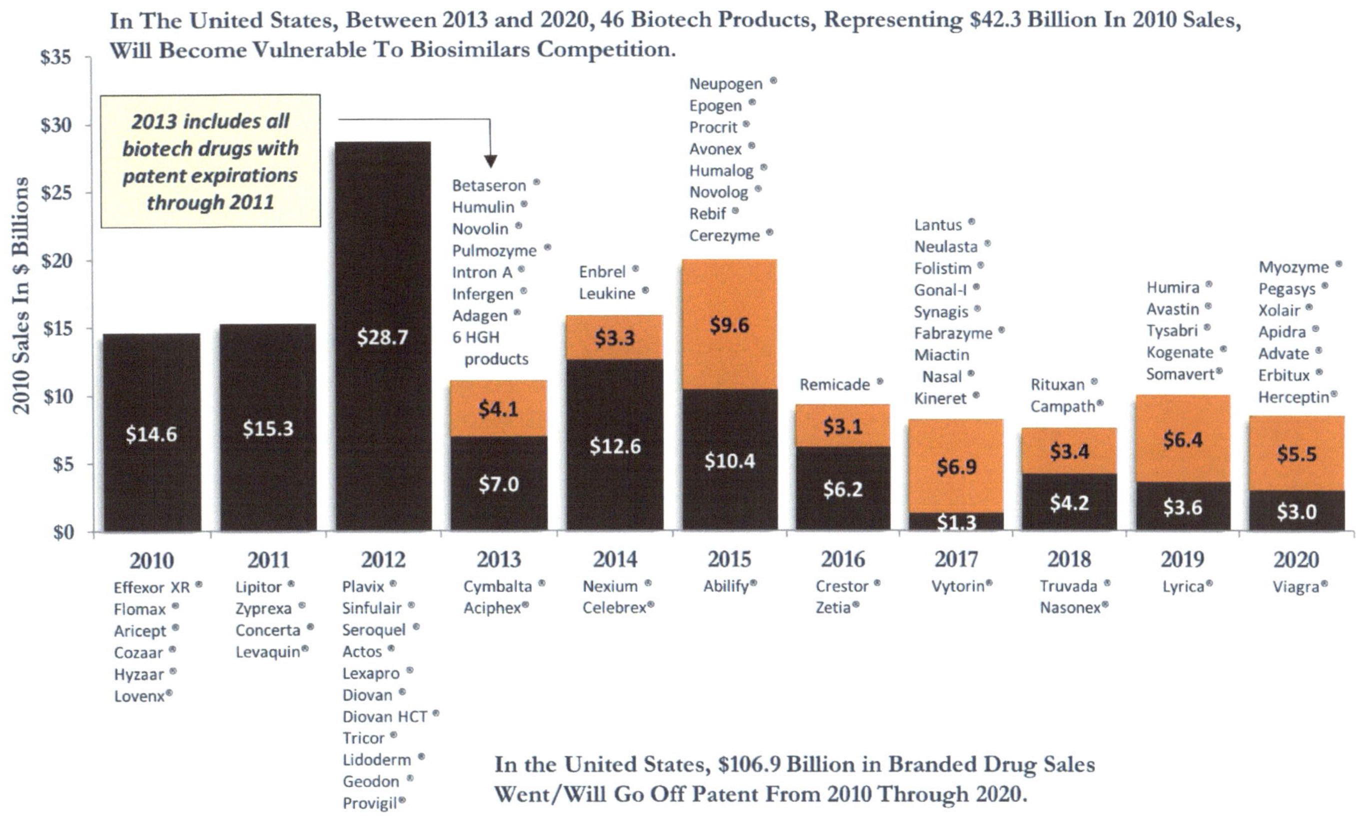

Sources: Prepared by MMC International. U.S. drug spend estimates based upon 2009 IMS Health data and manufacturer reported U.S. sales or a percent of manufacturer reported worldwide annual sales. Market availability of biosimilars based on expected patent expiration dates current as of November 2010 plus two years. Brand patent expiration dates were current as of December 2010. Changes may occur to dates due to litigation and patent challenges.

R&D will be transformed between 2012 and 2020 - and a new more productive model will emerge.

Two R&D indicators point toward a maturing and re-emerging pharmaceutical industry. As a technology hits its productivity limits, the cost of R&D per new product increases while the number of new products coming to market decreases. As the technology matures, the easiest products have been developed and the remaining products are increasingly more challenging/complex to develop. This continues until a new technology allows greater productivity which in turn redefines and revitalizes the maturing industry and replaces the old technology base. These trends are endemic of the transition which the pharmaceutical industry is undergoing. According to the Pharmaceutical R&D Factbook, compiled by CMR International, a Thomson Reuters business, drug success rates continued to show declining trends over the past decade. There were 55 Phase III drug terminations during the 2008 to 2010 period, more than double the number of terminations from 2005 to 2007. In addition, the number of drugs entering Phase III clinical trials fell by 55 percent in 2010. The complexity of new products demands more efficient patient targeting and R&D investigator and clinical operations. As a result, traditional pharmaceutical companies, which are represented by PhRMA (the Pharmaceutical Research and Manufacturers of America), began reducing their combined R&D investments in 2008, from a peak $47.9 billion in 2007 to $45.8 billion in 2009. This was more than offset by increasing investments in R&D by biotechnology companies.

Pharmaceuticals
Private and Public R&D Spending In $ Billions

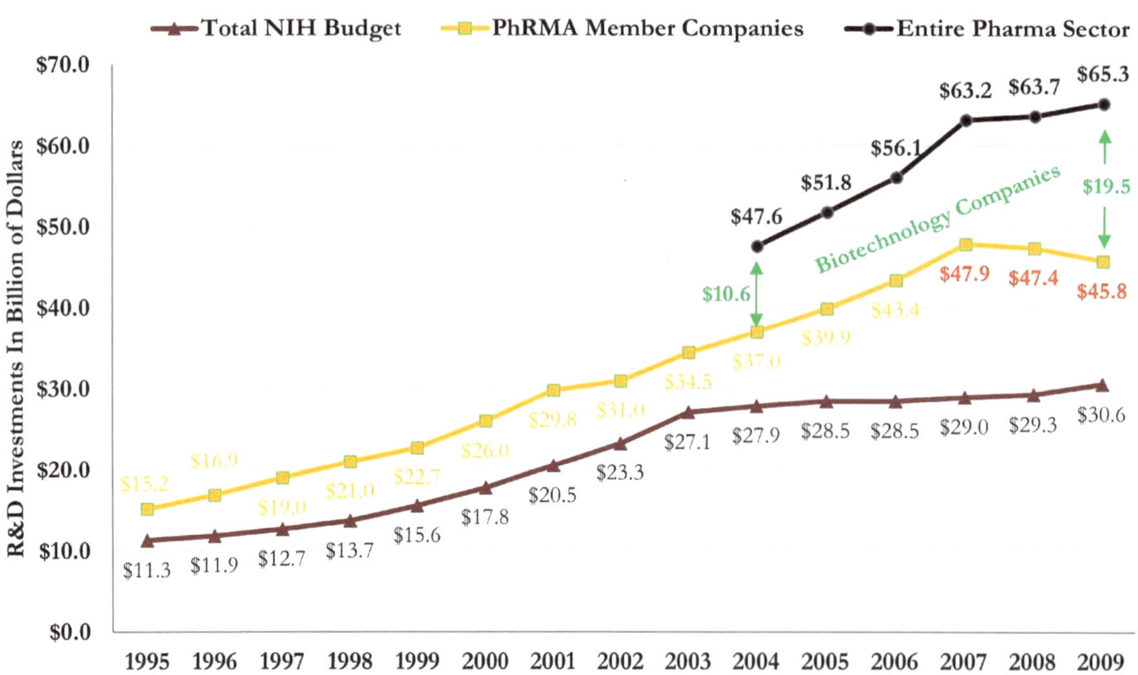

Source: Burrill & Company, PhRMA, NIH Office of Budget.

R&D and the regulatory approval process are expected to be redefined over the next few years.

The status quo is no longer an option. The limited number of remaining licensing, mergers and acquisitions opportunities can no longer supply the requisite products needed to sustain all the large pharmaceutical companies. Small molecule chemicals have reached their technology limitation. To survive, pharmaceutical companies have to innovate to increase their R&D productivity. The evolving R&D paradigm is toward niche drugs complemented by biomarkers which will be utilized to treat smaller identifiable reactive patient populations. The development time for these types of drugs can be significantly decreased via the utilization of: 1) new drug target identification tools (genomic and other databases, data mining software, biological modeling, etc.), 2) biomarkers to identify patients that will favorably respond to the drug, 3) combined clinical trial phases that will compress the clinical trial timeline, 4) utilization of significantly smaller reactive (identified using biomarker testing) clinical trial populations, and 5) a drug approval process that will limit the clinical trial to patients reactive to a specific biomarker – followed by post-marketing surveillance to insure the product's ongoing clinical safety. The Food and Drug administration has committed to work to make changes in the drug approval process to accommodate the changing research and development paradigm. Screening and predictive diagnostics and biomarkers will become more commonplace by 2020. The result should be: 1) shorter drug target identification and development times, 2) an increase in the number of products going into late stage clinical trials during the 2012 to 2020 timeframe, and 3) a growing number of new and novel products being approved during this timeframe. The approval of Zelboraf® is an example of this new process. It took Roche five years from Phase 1 to approval.

The United States Drug Approval Process Can Be Compressed
From 9.5 To 15 Years Down To Less Than Seven Years
Extracting Hundreds Of Millions Of Dollars From A Product's Development Cost

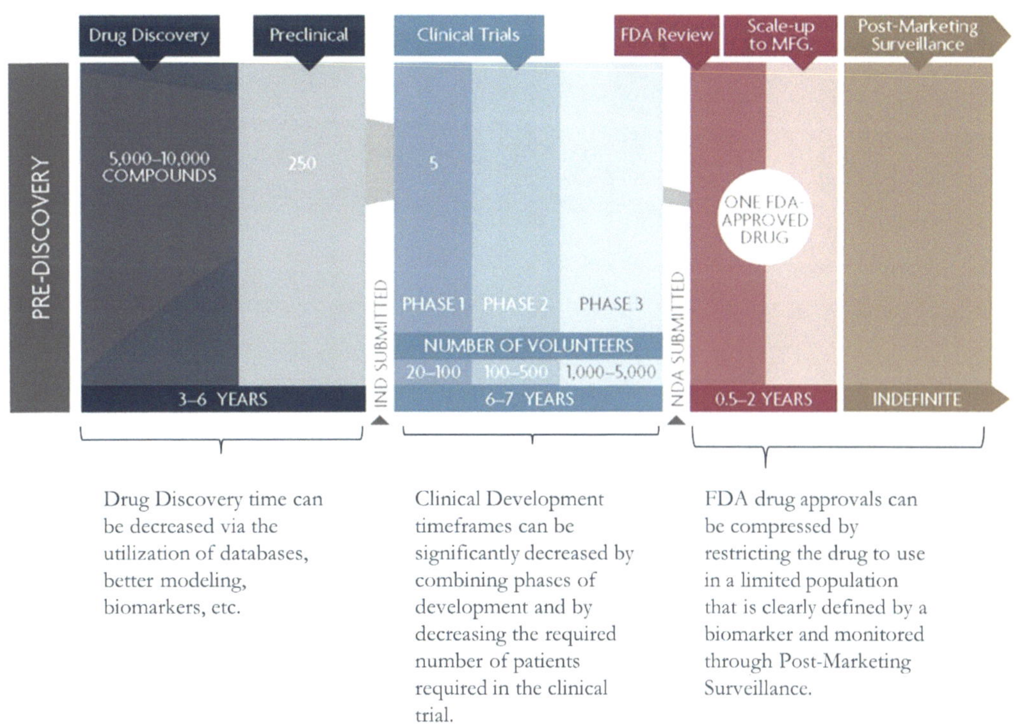

Sources: MMC International and PhRMA (traditional development cycle chart).

Persistence and compliance with prescriptions will drive value, sales and pharmaceutical profitability.

Failure to prescribe the indicated treatment occurs up to half the time in the United States. Adherence to long-term therapy for chronic illnesses in developed countries averages 50 percent. In 2010, according to CVS/Caremark, fewer than 40 percent of maintenance prescriptions were refilled on time and 31% of original maintenance prescriptions were never refilled. For every 100 prescriptions written only 15 percent to 20 percent are refilled as prescribed. Yet this is occurring in the face of overpowering evidence that using medications as recommended decreases adverse events, hospitalizations and deaths. Another problem is underdiagnosis. As an example, uncontrolled diabetes can lead to kidney failure, amputations, and stroke. If untreated hypertensive patients received recommended medications, hospitalizations would decrease by 49.6 percent, from 833,000 down to 420,000 per year – annual premature deaths would decrease by 89,000. Managing the outcome of the patient by providing proper screening, prescribing and prescription compliance and persistence would save the U.S. healthcare system billions of dollars over and above the incremental medication and program costs. Sharing in the extraction of these needless costs is one of the areas of focus for pharmaceutical manufacturers and payers alike. The Patient-Centered Outcomes Research Institute (PCORI), created in 2010 by the Patient Protection and Affordable Care Act (PPACA), is a private, non-profit entity. The Institute will spearhead efforts to prioritize and fund comparative effectiveness research (CER) using a largely stakeholder-driven process. This initiative builds upon the strong foundation laid in 2009 by the $1.1 billion in funding for CER in the American Recovery and Reinvestment Act (ARRA). Utilization of health technology assessments to quantify the value of a specific product or drug offering (product plus value-added services) will facilitate the transition to an outcomes, value-based pricing system. Different models will emerge between 2012 and 2020. The formulas used for reimbursement will be therapy and product specific. Health technology assessment (HTA) will increasingly drive reimbursement for new products. To avoid extreme price pressure and/or the risk of not being approved for reimbursement will continue to push the risk/reward model, given the new R&D paradigm, towards new and novel innovative therapies and away from me-too follow-on drugs. This will serve to further reinvigorate the pharmaceutical industry.

Drug reimbursement will dictate the speed and direction of the pharmaceutical industry change.

Pharmaceutical companies are well positioned to extract costs from the healthcare system. The linkage between benefits, risks, product and treatment/therapy cost is getting stronger. The years of expansion and profitability fueled by being able to launch any new product, e.g., me-too products, is quickly giving way to a cost-justified reimbursement era where not all products will be reimbursable. New products will increasingly require proof of substantial incremental clinical and/or cost benefits. The biggest benefit for chronic care medications (versus episodic medications), for payers and pharmaceutical companies alike, is proper prescribing and patient persistence and compliance. This requires: 1) physician education to insure physicians know how to use the product correctly, 2) patient screening to identify candidate patients and those patients which would benefit from the drug, 3) an objective measure that indicates the drug is working and that the patient is in compliance with the therapy, 4) outcomes-based provider reimbursement for maintaining patients within accepted outcomes ranges which indicate proper disease management, and 5) coordination with patient educators, counselors, disease patient organizations/groups, prescribed treatment protocols, and disease management companies. Only two organizations in United States healthcare have the ability to roll out such a program on a uniform and national basis, health insurers and pharmaceutical companies. Pharmaceutical companies are the only organizations that are truly national and that are capable of uniformly educating physicians and all related stakeholders. In addition, since the pharmaceutical company developed the drug and/or is marketing the drug, that company is the most knowledgeable about the disease, therapy, and how the drug fits in clinical management. The transition by pharmaceutical companies from drugs to outcomes will require reimbursement changes and alliances. The entities that will have to be engaged prior to launching a new drug will explode. New players, that influence prescribing and reimbursement, will have to be engaged to achieve an optimal patient outcome. Innovation will redefine industry norms. The shift to outcomes will improve persistence and compliance and thereby increase U.S. sales. Delivering an outcome rather than a drug justifies higher drug pricing. The opportunities will be drug, product portfolio, and company specific. The transition from traditional pharmaceuticals to selling outcomes will revitalize a newly defined, opportunity rich marketplace. However, many companies will have to bridge a challenging period between 2012 and 2016, when they will lose patent protection for major drugs, in order to prosper in the new industry. Some will not survive.

Samples of Non-Traditional Partners

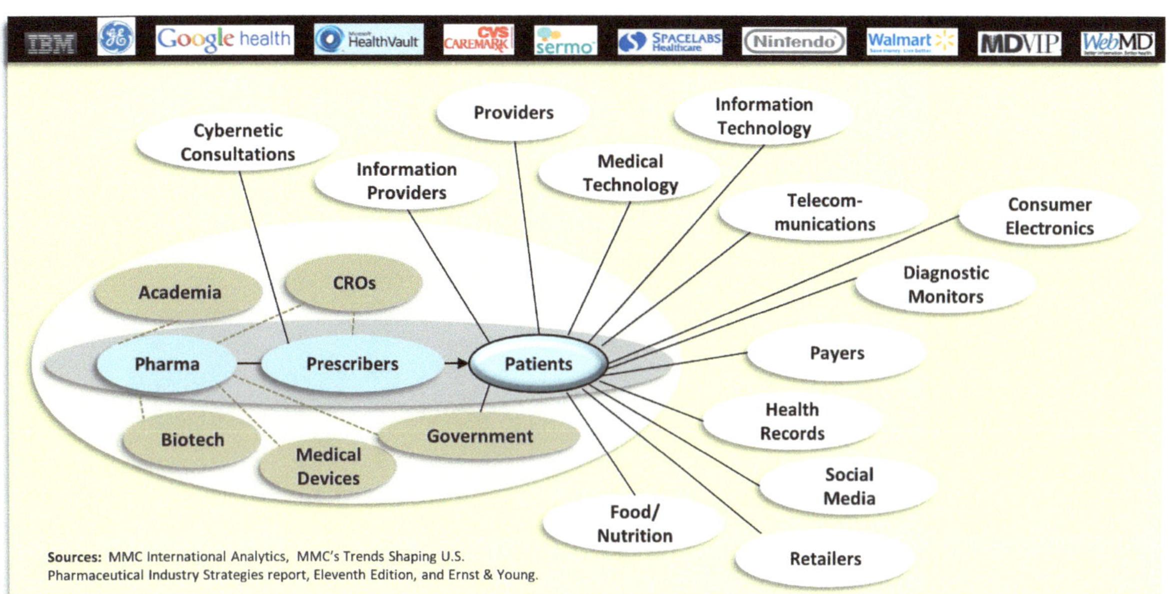

The "outcome value" of the total offering may become an entry barrier to generic competition. It will be the cost/value of the outcome, not the cost of the drug. Disease management, compliance, and persistence will grow in importance. For many products, they will become a core of the results/outcome offering. Partnering with non-traditional partners will become a differentiating core competency that will need to be integrated into the drug development process.

Branded companies are moving into generics to protect their franchises when protection expires.

The rapid market share erosion, over 98 percent of a brand's volume within 12 months after protection expires, explains why branded companies are moving into generics or developing strategies to retain share even at generic or lower prices after their products lose protection (patent, patent term extension, Orphan Drug, etc.). Simply stated, it maximizes shareholder returns.

Market Share Erosion
Within 12 Months Of Post-Protection Expiration

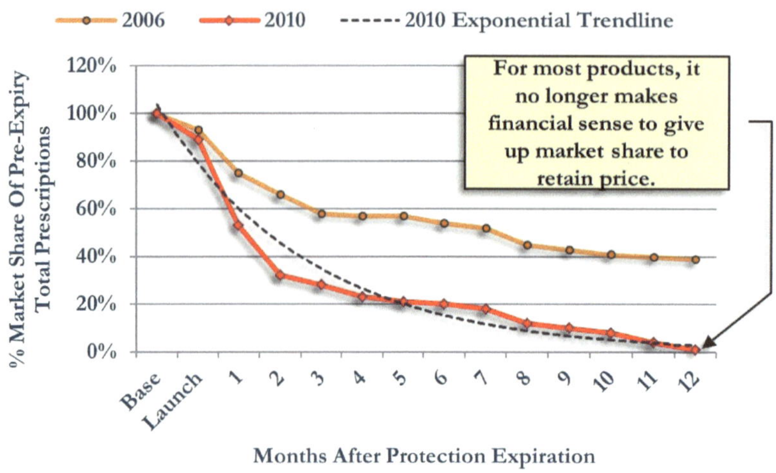

Sources: IMS National Prescription Audit Plus, Feb. 2011 and MMC International.

Once the returns of maintaining brand share, in light of generics competition, equals or is greater than maintaining a premium price for the brand, then a fundamental power shift occurs. The brand, with its inherent scale economies for the particular product, is in the position to maintain market share as long as it maintains the position of the low-cost manufacturer and as long as it is willing to decrease price to maintain share.

Between 2012 and 2020, generics manufacturers can expect to encounter stiff price competition from originators who will increasingly be willing to drop their prices to maintain share. For any given product, pricing instability in light of generics will continue until the relationship between manufacturers makes it too expensive for the number two and the rest of the manufacturers to invest in strategies to increase product share.

Sources: MMC Insights, Two Seminal Events Signal Transformation of the Pharmaceutical Industry by Edmund L. Valentine, 2006, and MMC International.

The U.S. generics market is only about 40% of the way toward becoming a mature market.

While innovative/branded pharmaceuticals are in the mature phase of their lifecycle, the U.S. generics market is only about 40% of the way toward becoming a fully mature market – although the global generics industry is moving toward an oligopoly. The key challenge for generics companies will be changing marketplace norms as pharmaceutical companies strive to retain their market shares. The industry is sufficiently mature that the largest generics drug companies, with their increasing free cash flows, are well positioned to acquire biotechnology and small pharmaceutical companies. Slowly the industry is coming together into a pharmaceutical care industry rather than separate pharmaceutical, biotechnology and generics companies. It also affords them the ability to develop select innovative products, biosimilar/bioequivalent agents, and to begin positioning themselves to thrive in the new, emerging pharmaceutical care industry. The major generics companies are well positioned to capitalize on the changing industry as they have low-cost manufacturing, predictable free cash flows, deep generics pipelines, and increasing global scale.

Top 10 Generics Companies Relative Market Share
Dispensed Generic Prescriptions

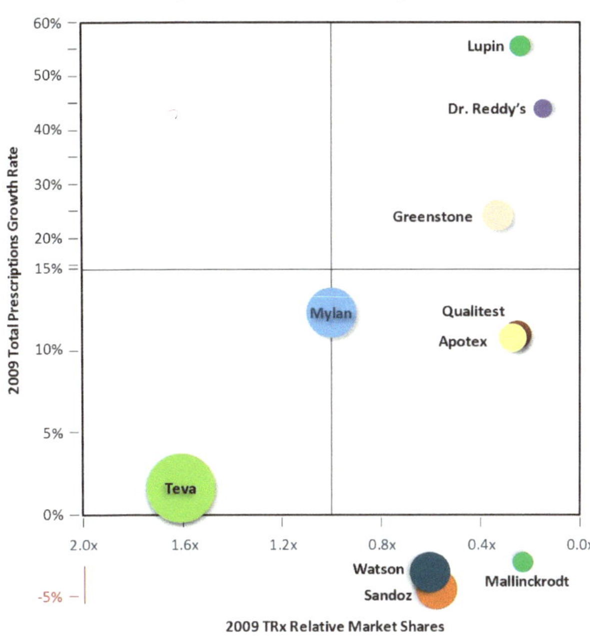

Sources: MMC International and IMS Health, MIDAS, MAT Sept. 2009 data.

For the U.S. generics market to become mature, the market leader would have to increase its market share to about 57% and the number two company to around 28%.

Dispensed Generic Rxs By Leading Companies

	TRxs (Millions)	Market Share	2009 Growth
U.S INDUSTRY	**2,568**		**7.5%**
1. Teva	556	21.7%	1.7%
2. Mylan	336	13.1%	12.3%
3. Watson	184	7.2%	-4.1%
4. Sandoz (Novartis)	176	6.9%	-5.5%
5. Greenstone (Pfizer)	109	4.2%	24.4%
6. Apotex	99	3.9%	11.2%
7. Qualitest	96	3.7%	11.5%
8. Lupin	90	3.5%	56.0%
9. Mallinckrodt	89	3.5%	-3.4%
10. Dr. Reddy	70	2.7%	43.6%
Top 10	**1,805**	**70.3%**	**7.1%**

Source: IMS Health, MIDAS, MAT Sept. 2009.

The largest companies are the best positioned to capitalize on change.

The medium (those over $500 million in sales) and big (over $5 billion) pharmaceutical, biotechnology and/or generics companies are the best positioned to morph their companies to capitalize upon the changing pharmaceutical industry between 2012 and 2020. How the industry evolves is dependent upon legislation, regulations, reimbursement, scientific progress, and how different companies innovate to capture competitive advantage. The only certainties between 2012 and 2020 are that the industry will change and that the industry will be redefined. Some companies will be carved up; others will be acquired, merged or driven out of business. The companies that succeed will be strategically driven. They will be handsomely rewarded. They will create considerable corporate and shareholder wealth.

Top 50 2010 Companies Ranked By Healthcare Revenue

Rank 2010	Company	Headquarters	Healthcare Revenues (in $ Billions)	Pharma-ceuticals	Generics	Biologics	Biopharma	Vaccines	Diagnostics	Medical Devices	OTC	Animal Health	Nutri-tionals
1	Pfizer Inc.	New York, NY	67.8	X			X	X			X	X	X
2	Johnson & Johnson	New Brunswick, NJ	61.6	X					X	X	X		
3	Novartis AG	Basel, Switzerland	50.6	X	X			X	X		X	X	
4	Merck & Co.	Whitehouse Station, NJ	46.0	X		X		X			X	X	
5	F. Hoffmann-La Roche Ltd.	Basel, Switzerland	45.5	X			X		X				
6	GlaxoSmithKline Plc.	Brentford, United Kingdom	43.9	X				X			X		
7	Sanofi SA	Paris, France	40.3	X	X			X			X	X	
8	Abbott Laboratories	Abbott Park, IL	35.2	X		X	X	X	X	X	X	X	X
9	AstraZeneca Plc.	London, United Kingdom	33.3	X			X						
10	Eli Lilly and Co.	Indianapolis, IN	23.1	X								X	
11	Bayer AG	Leverkusen, Germany	22.4	X		X				X	X	X	
12	Bristol-Myers Squibb Co.	New York, NY	19.5	X			X						
13	Boehringer Ingelheim GmbH	Ingelheim, Germany	16.7	X			X				X	X	
14	Takeda Pharmaceutical Co.	Osaka	16.3	X							X		
15	Teva Pharmaceutical Industries Ltd.	Petach Tikva, Israel	16.1	X	X		X					X	
16	Amgen Inc.	Thousand Oaks, CA	15.1	X			X						
17	Baxter International Inc.	Deerfield, IL	12.8	X		X				X			
18	Otsuka Holdings Co.	Tokyo	12.5	X							X		
19	Daiichi Sankyo Co.	Tokyo	11.8	X	X						X		
20	Astellas Pharma Inc.	Tokyo	11.7	X									
21	Novo Nordisk AS	Bagsvaerd, Denmark	10.8	X			X				X		
22	Eisai Co.	Tokyo	9.1	X					X		X		
23	Merck KGaA	Darmstadt, Germany	8.0	X			X				X		
24	Gilead Sciences Inc.	Foster City , CA	7.9				X						
25	Allergan Inc.	Irvine, CA	4.9	X		X				X			
26	Mitsubishi Tanabe Pharma Corp.	Osaka	4.9	X							X		
27	Biogen Idec Inc.	Weston, MA	4.7				X						
28	Mylan Inc.	Canonsburg, PA	4.5	X	X								
29	CSL Ltd.	Parkville	4.4	X		X		X	X				
30	Forest Laboratories Inc.	New York, NY	4.4	X							X		
31	Chugai Pharmaceutical Co.	Tokyo	4.3	X									
32	UCB SA	Brussels, Belgium	4.3				X						
33	Nycomed Group	Zurich, Switzerland	4.2	X							X		
34	Dainippon Sumitomo Pharma Co.	Osaka	4.1	X					X			X	
35	Hospira Inc.	Lake Forest, IL	3.9		X					X			
36	Celgene Corp.	Summit, NJ	3.6				X						
37	Watson Pharmaceuticals Inc.	Parsippany, NJ	3.6	X	X								
38	Shire Plc.	Dublin, Ireland	3.5	X			X						
39	Shionogi & Co.	Osaka	3.5	X					X		X		
40	Taisho Pharmaceutical Co.	Tokyo	3.3	X							X		X
41	Warner Chilcott Plc.	Dublin, Ireland	3.0	X									
42	Cephalon Inc.	Frazer, PA	2.8				X						
43	H. Lundbeck AS	Copenhagen, Denmark	2.6	X									
44	Kyowa Hakko Kirin Co.	Tokyo	2.4	X									
45	Stada Arzneimittel AG	Bad Vilbel, Germany	2.2	X	X								
46	Ranbaxy Laboratories Ltd.	Gurgaon (Haryana)	1.9	X	X								
47	Actelion Pharmaceuticals Ltd.	Allschwil, Switzerland	1.8				X						
48	Endo Pharmaceuticals Holdings Inc.	Chadds Ford, PA	1.7	X	X								
49	Teijin Ltd.	Osaka	1.7	X									
50	Ono Pharmaceutical Co.	Osaka	1.7	X					X				

Sources: MMC International, MedAdNews, and company reports.

19 IN VITRO DIAGNOSTICS

In vitro diagnostics is an opportunity rich industry which will be transformed between 2012 and 2020.

The $44 billion global in vitro diagnostics industry (IVD), a global growth business thirty-five percent of the way to becoming a mature market, is well positioned to capitalize on industry change. Diagnostics account for about two percent of healthcare expenditures but are instrumental in seventy percent of clinical decisions. Genomics and new technologies, instrumentation and related software are resulting in an increasing number of tests with improving sensitivity and specificity. New products will include stand-alone tests, testing systems, companion tests for a specific drug/drugs, and device-diagnostic and device-diagnostic-drug combinations. All are expected to benefit from health technology assessments which will demonstrate the cost effectiveness and clinical benefits of utilizing a specific test/diagnostic system in specified therapies. The utilization of electronic health records, prescribed treatment protocols, requirements for outcomes measurements, and disease management will assist in speeding adoption and utilization of the new tests. Products range from high-volume, low-cost, price-driven generic tests to an emerging group of novel tests that have the potential to rival the drug prices and sales volumes of some biotechnology drugs. Diagnostics are required to: 1) screen populations for disease, 2) monitor health, 3) establish the prognosis for a specific disease or condition, 4) predict a person's probability of getting a specific disease or developing a specific condition, 5) identify individuals that will respond to a particular drug, 6) identify those individuals that may have an adverse reaction(s) to a medication, and 7) monitor compliance with therapy/treatment. In academia and drug development, diagnostics are used to speed the process of identifying and validating potential targets for drug development. The diagnostics industry will undergo significant change, growth, and further consolidation between 2012 and 2020 – creating corporate and personal wealth.

In Vitro Diagnostics Lifecycle

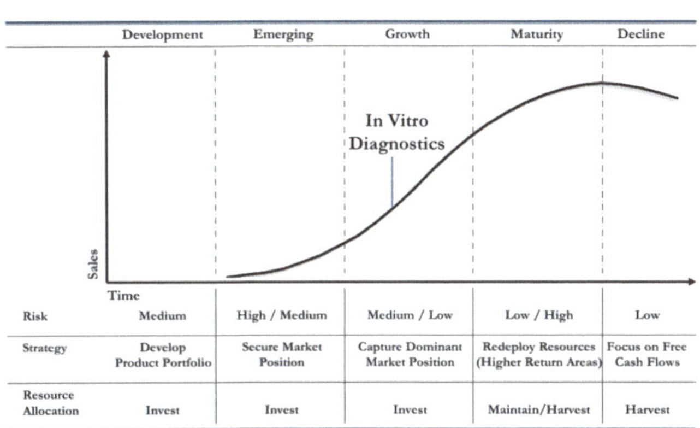

Source: MMC International.

Global In Vitro Diagnostics Major Competitors' Relative Market Shares

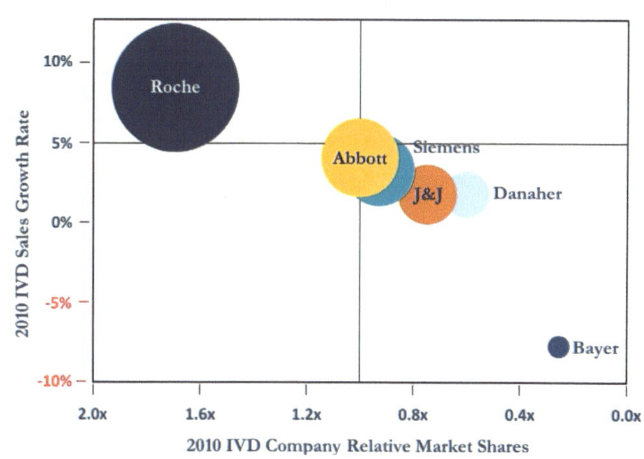

Source: MMC International and Roche Investor Day Presentations, 2010.

The traditional high-volume tests IVD business favors large competitors.

Unlike branded pharmaceuticals, which depend on patent/exclusivity protection for success, the traditional high-volume IVD market depends on the breadth of the test portfolio tied to proprietary testing systems to acquire and retain market share. Since a myriad of tests will continue to be introduced, the major IVD competitors have focused on the development and placement of modular systems that accommodate capacity expansion via the addition of system modules. Their focus is on automation, workflow integration within the lab and the provider network, and lab information management. Generally, these systems are closed (other manufacturers' tests cannot not be used in the system) – making this a razor/razor blade market. The larger competitors use price bundling for their tests and systems offerings to create barriers to entry. Typically, system contracts span a number of years; making displacement especially challenging. In turn, major competitors are in an excellent position to partner with smaller companies focused upon a test or a few tests if those tests require processing by clinical laboratories, hospitals, clinics or in physicians' offices – versus a specialty laboratory. They are also in an excellent position to consolidate the market as it begins to mature.

Sample IVD Commercial Lab And Hospital Systems

Roche's In Vitro Diagnostics System

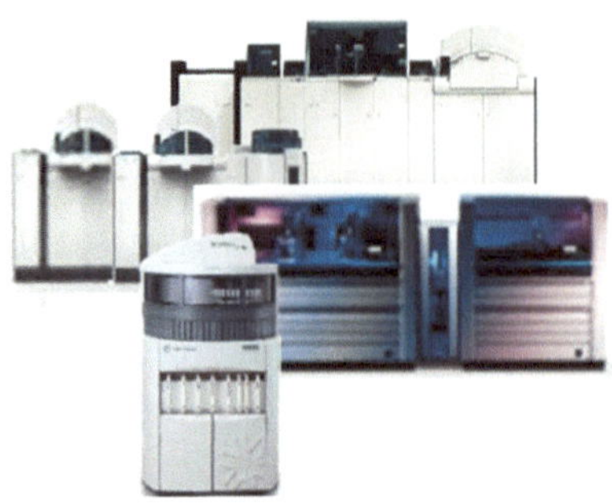

Ortho Clinical Diagnostics' (J&J) In Vitro Diagnostics System

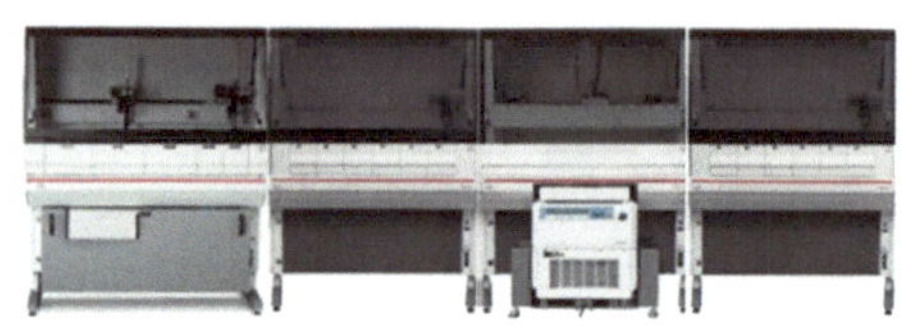

Abbott's In Vitro Diagnostics System

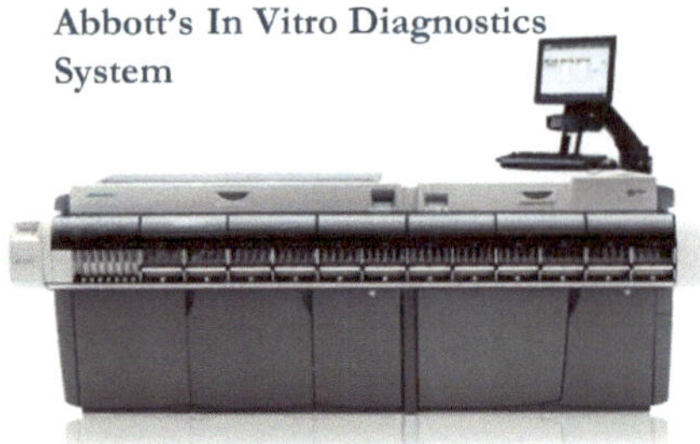

Abbott's In Vitro Molecular Diagnostics System

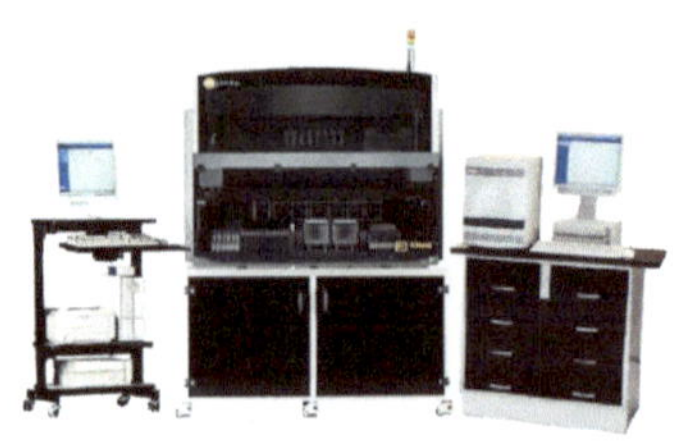

Siemens' In Vitro Diagnostics System

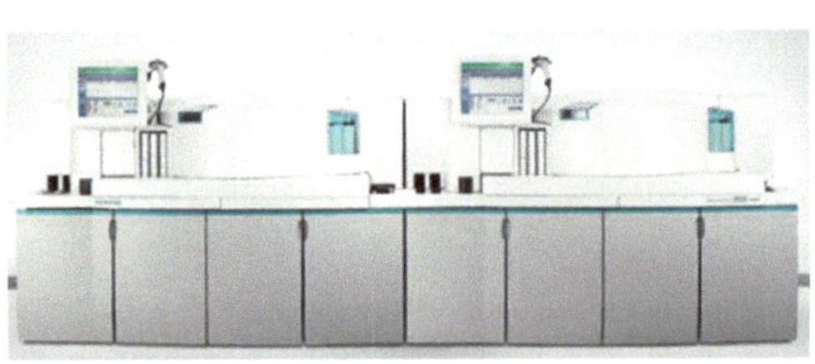

Danaher's In Vitro Diagnostics System

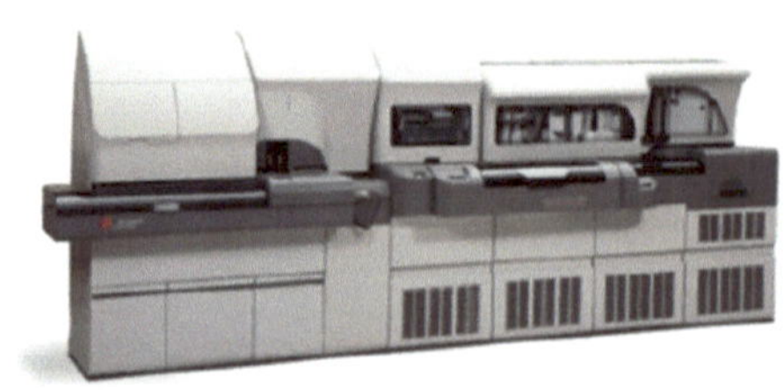

The IVD market is made up of a number of customer and testing segments- representing opportunities.

The IVD market is comprised of a myriad of market segments. The market can be segmented by the type of diagnostics: applied science (academia and pharmaceuticals), molecular diagnostics (molecular laboratories and blood screening), tissue diagnostics (pathology laboratory), professional diagnostics (central laboratory, emergency room, intensive care units, and doctors' offices), and home diagnostics (patients). Customers range from commercial laboratories and hospitals for clinical systems to physicians' offices, health clinics, and home for point-of-care diagnostics. There are opportunities in all segments. The segments that represent the highest rates of growth include: tissue diagnostics, molecular diagnostics, point-of-care diagnostics, biomarkers (Theranostics), home/OTC diagnostics, and the emerging market for predictive diagnostics.

Sample Point of Care (PoC) Diagnostic Systems

Siemens' Stratus CS
Acute Care Diagnostic System

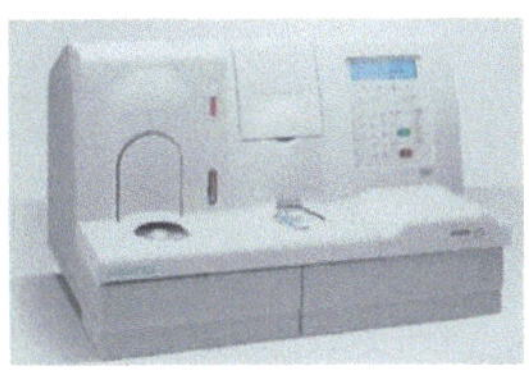

Abbott's iStat®
PoC Diagnostics System

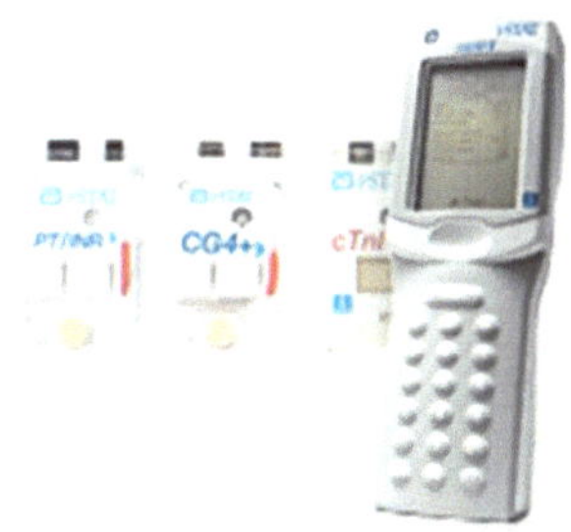

Samples Of Various PoC Tests/Systems

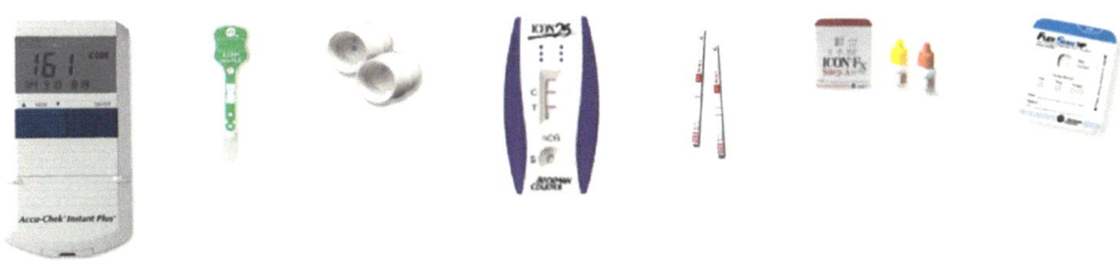

Roche's Chemstrip®
Criterion II PoC Analyzer

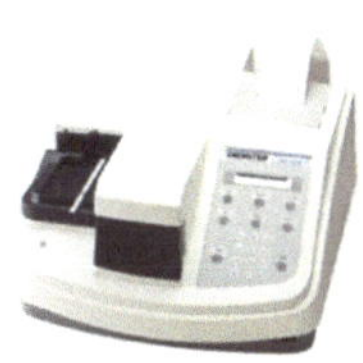

Intellectual property is widely available for most IVD tests – this is changing for high-value assays.

Historically, diagnostic companies focused on testing efficacy. More recently, this has expanded to include medical value. The main focus by 2020 will be on proven medical value, on translational diagnostics. Ideally, payers and providers not only want a particular measure; they also want to know what it means, i.e., what to do from a patient treatment perspective. To answer what it means requires costly clinical trials and clinical data to translate the diagnostic into therapy. This is more akin to the pharmaceutical model where intellectual property is protected and required for profitability. This also requires a shift to value reimbursement. This process has already begun. As an example, the Oncotype DX test first received a positive Medicare coverage decision in 2004 for breast cancer and on September 18, 2011 for colon cancer. It has a list price of $3,280.00. Oncotype DX's global annual market potential for use in three cancers, breast, colon and prostate, is 1.2 million patients, $3.9 billion. The growing number of potential targets, the growing demand for biomarkers, the potential market for prognostic testing to enable disease prevention before the disease or condition materializes, the potential market size for individual IVD tests, etc., has, is and will result in the creation of new companies to develop these higher margin, large potential market, types of assays.

Demonstrating Clinical Utility and Health Economic Benefit Results in a Higher Reimbursement And Greater Returns For The Innovator

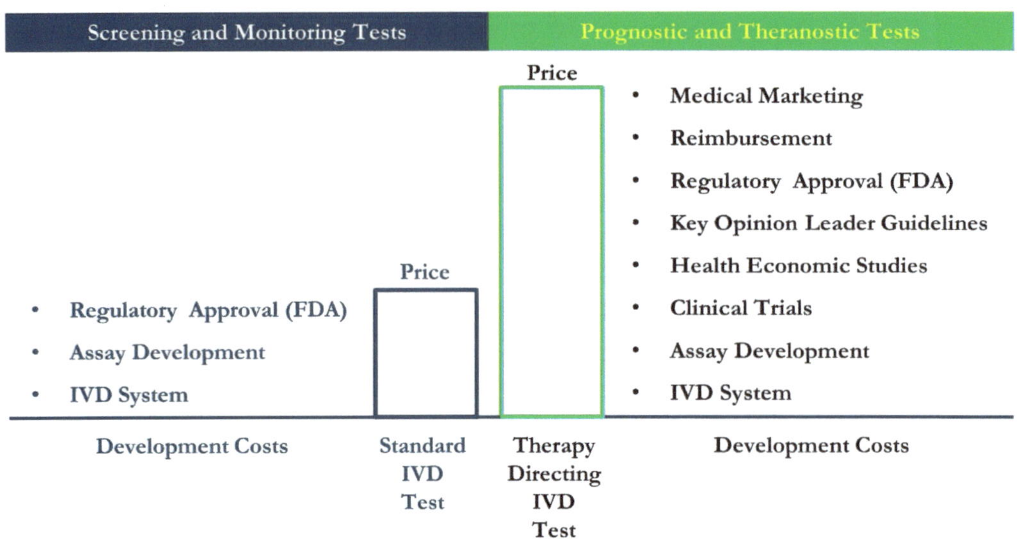

Source: MMC International.

Genomics is in the early stages of redefining the in vitro diagnostics industry.

Genomics is in the early stages of redefining the IVD marketplace from providing values to translational diagnostics. This is akin to the emergence of biotechnology when the pharmaceutical industry was in its growth phase. Genomics is enabling the creation of start-up companies around proprietary advanced molecular tests designed to assist in cost-effectively managing patient treatment. As an example, only three- to four-percent of patients with early stage colon cancer react to chemotherapy; ninety percent of prostate cancer patients do well without surgery; and women with breast cancer have been treated with chemotherapy even though only a small subset may benefit. Genomic Health, Inc., founded in 2000, introduced the first gene expression test in 2004 to address these issues. Oncotype DX is a $3,280.00 proprietary test that cost effectively addresses these issues. It predicts the likelihood of benefit from chemotherapy in estrogen receptor-positive, lymph node negative breast cancer patients. This information is valuable in determining if a patient can safely avoid the cytotoxic effects and high costs of chemotherapy. Prior to the utilization of Oncotype DX, sixty-two percent of candidate breast cancer patients were recommended for chemotherapy. The number decreased to thirty-five percent of candidate breast cancer patients after screening them with Oncotype DX, a thirty-seven percent change in the course of treatment. Oncotype DX also predicts the likelihood of reoccurrence of Stage II colon cancer, allowing doctors to pursue more aggressive therapy for these patients and avoiding expensive unneeded care for the majority of patients. Late stage clinical trials indicate that Oncotype DX will also identify the ten percent of prostate cancer patients with aggressive cancer that require surgery – avoiding the cost of surgery and the side effects for the ninety percent of patients that do not require surgery. Genomic Health has a global price for Oncotype DX and processes assays received from around the world – from sixty countries as of 2011, in its central laboratory. Historically, diagnostic testing has been done in local or national laboratories; not in a single, global laboratory. Genomic Health has proven the viability of a new diagnostic model based upon the development of a single, novel, protected, high-value diagnostic that improves care and reduces needless care – Genomic Health turned profitable in 2010.

295 Genes Predict Prostate Cancer Clinical Recurrence (Unadjusted P<0.05)

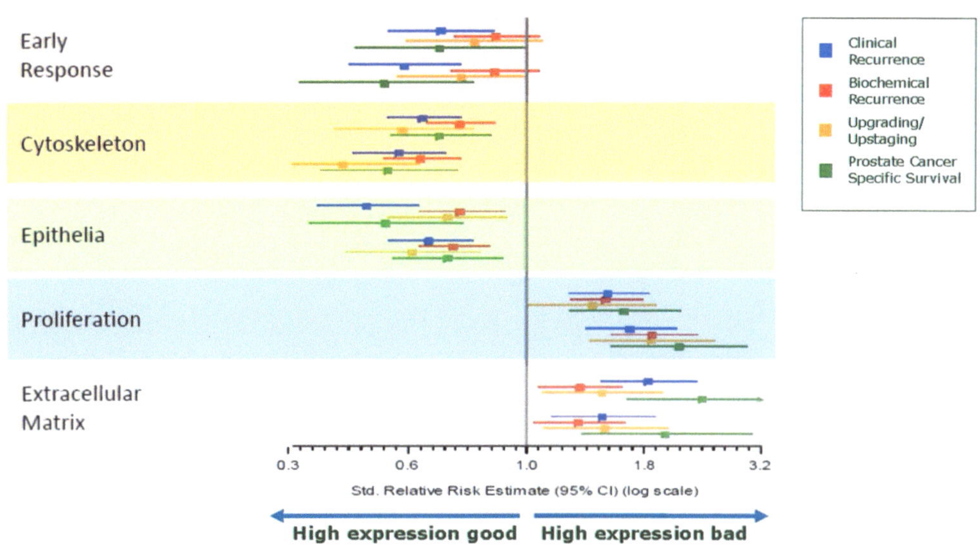

Source: Genomic Health, Large Prostate Study Reveals Hundreds of Genes Strongly Associated With Clinical Recurrence, Investor Presentation, November 1, 2011.

The value of companion diagnostics requires pharmaceutical companies to access IVD technologies.

Most drugs have been developed based on the disease, not on the underlying molecular causes. This, in part, explains why half of the prescription drugs taken by patients fail to achieve the desired clinical outcome. In addition, the majority of drugs fail in clinical trials due to efficacy. This can be overcome through the development of targeted therapies which require testing of defined populations to insure that the drug's mechanism of action will have the desired therapeutic effect. Personalized medicine (i.e., patient stratification) reduces the total potential patient pool, versus how drugs were previously developed, for a defined patient population. The offset will be: 1) lower development costs due to fewer patients required in clinical trials and fewer drug failures in advanced stages of drug development, 2) shorter development timelines due to fewer patients required for clinical trials, 3) faster market penetration due to the ability to define reactive patients and an increasing number of reimbursement schemes that require/will require physicians to follow prescribed treatment protocols for specific diseases/conditions, 4) increased market share due to the specificity/personalized bases of treatment, and 5) higher prices/pricing stability due to pricing based upon the total cost of patient care/outcome rather than on the price of the drug.

Benefits From Personalized Healthcare
Rewards Both Pharmaceutical and Diagnostics Companies

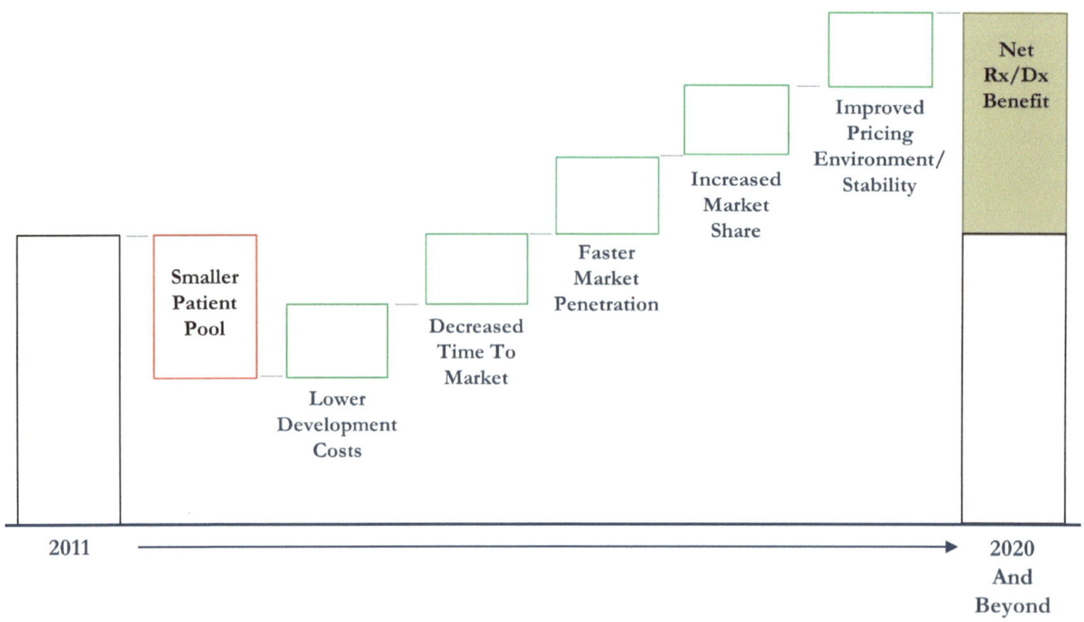

Source: MMC International.

Pharmaceutical and diagnostics deal making will increase between 2012 and 2020.

By 2020 drug-diagnostic co-development is expected to become routine for drugs for which biomarkers are relevant. In addition, most leading pharmaceutical companies will have incorporated significant diagnostics capabilities in-house. The development of diagnostics to set clinical direction and the potential of being able to protect the intellectual property of the tests; along with the changing reimbursement for translational tests, will potentially make diagnostics more attractive to pharmaceutical companies. Pharmaceutical companies have three options to access diagnostics (Dx) technologies: 1) external partnerships/licensing, 2) acquire diagnostics businesses, and/or 3) for companies with existing diagnostic operations, cooperation between the pharmaceutical and diagnostics operations. The only certainty is that a number of different models will emerge and that demand for companion diagnostics will increase. The best positioned companies to capitalize on diagnostics industry growth are the market leaders in each of the respective diagnostic industry segments.

In Vitro Diagnostics Companies Portfolio Breadth By Market Segment

Breadth of Portfolio Offering From Narrow To Broad: ◔ ◑ ◕ ●

	IVD Market Leaders						Examples Of Other IVD Companies					
IVD Market Segments	Roche	Abbott	Siemens	Johnson & Johnson	Danaher*	bioMerieux	Alere	Beckton Dickinson	Cepheld	Gen-Probe	Novartis	Qiagen
Clinical Chemistry	●	●	●	◑	◕							
Immunoassays	●	●	●	◑	◕	◑	◔					
Hematology	◑	◕	◕		●							
Coagulation	◑		●		◑							
Urinalysis	●	●										
Point of Care	◕	◑	◑		◔	◔	●					
Automation	◕	◕	◔	◔	◕							
Virology	●	●	●			◑		◔	◔	◔		◑
Blood Screening	●										●	
Human papillomavirus (HPV)	●	◑				◔				◔		●
Chlamydia Trachomatis and Neisseria Gonorrhea (CT/NG)	●	●	◔					●		●		◑
Microbiology	◑	◔				◔		●	●	◑		◔
Genomics & Oncology	◑	◑							◔	◑		◑
IVD 2010 Market Share	20%	12%	11%	9%	7%	3%						

* Danaher market share based upon Beckman Coulter's 2010 market share.

Note: The following pharmaceutical companies have diagnostic operations: Abbott, Bayer, Johnson & Johnson, Novartis, and Sanofi-Aventis.

There were 46 companion diagnostic deals done by pharmaceutical companies in 2009 through mid-2010: GlaxoSmithKline did 7, Pfizer 4, Roche 4, Bayer Schering 3, Bristol Myers Squibb 3, Eli Lilly 3, Merck & Co. 3, Novartis 3, Astellas (OSI) 2, AstraZeneca 2, Merck KGaA 2, and 10 companies entered into single deals.

The following were the most active diagnostic companies in companion diagnostics between 2009 and mid-2010: Qiagen with 5 deals, Almac 4, Roche 4, Abbott 3, Dako 3, MDxHealth 3, bioMerieux 2, DiaGenic 2, and Prometheus 2. There were 16 single company dealmakers.

20 MEDICAL DEVICES

Medical devices, an opportunity-rich market, will experience increasing consolidation through 2020.

The United States $106 billion (in 2011) medical devices industry is a maturing, opportunity-rich marketplace with over 6,000 companies selling in excess of 130,000 FDA approved products. The United States is: 1) the largest global medical devices market (about half of global sales), 2) the world's technological innovation leader, and 3) home to many of the world's leading medical device manufacturers, e.g., Johnson & Johnson, General Electric, Baxter, Covidien and Medtronic. Seven out of the world's top ten device manufacturers are United States headquartered companies. Devices range from basic supplies such as syringes, needles, bandages, implantable screws and blood pressure monitors through to anesthetic equipment, surgical instruments, heart pacemakers, hip prostheses, coronary stents, catheters, therapeutic and diagnostic X-ray equipment and MRI scanners. Products range from commodities to highly differentiated and patent-protected medical devices. Medical devices include in vitro diagnostic products (previously covered), certain electronic radiation emitting products with medical applications and claims, diagnostic ultrasound products, x-ray machines and medical lasers. Combination device/drug products include drug-eluting stents, drug/syringe combinations, drug/inhaler combinations, and implantable drug delivery devices. Continual glucose monitoring (CGM) devices are an example of a diagnostic/device combination product. The diagnostic/drug/device combination includes the glucose closed loop systems (artificial pancreas) in clinical trials. The systems are comprised of a CGM, an insulin pump and insulin. The attractiveness of medical devices was highlighted at the end of 2011 when both Abbott Laboratories and Covidien announced their intentions to spin off their pharmaceutical businesses to focus on medical devices to foster growth and improve stock valuations/performance - thereby increasing shareholder value. The period from 2012 to 2020 will be a period of innovation, consolidation and industry discontinuity as companies reposition themselves to maintain or improve their historic sales growth and/or profitability and valuations in the face of customer and competitive pressures. Medical devices are a global business that, for the most part, benefit from both economies of scale and shared economies of scale. Traditional marketplace rules will serve to shape competitive strategies. Discontinuities will result in changed industry norms during the 2012 to 2020 period and lead to strategic acquisitions/consolidation and new market entrants (e.g., electronic chip manufacturers, materials science companies, and healthcare information technology services, etc.). The only certainty is that the industry will be transformed by 2020 and that strategically-driven companies will prosper and create significant corporate as well as personal wealth. Many companies will be broken up, merged, acquired or driven out of business.

The medical device sales equation will shift between 2012 to 2020 – disrupting historic industry norms.

The main PPACA legislation impact on medical devices will be the migration in product/brand decision-making power from physicians to purchasing managers/medical administrators and patients. The shift will be especially severe for non-differentiated (generic) products and for substitutable products that will come under increasing pricing pressures. Medical device sales and marketing expenses can run as high as thirty or forty percent of revenues. The traditional sales and marketing model using intense, direct contact with physicians to influence product decisions is still warranted and profitable for differentiated products; but in others, it may not be. For this reason, the medical device firms are fine-tuning or completely transforming their sales and marketing models to reflect the migration to a bid and procurement model where the physician has limited or no influence. The effects of these changes can be illustrated by recent actions by Medtronic, which is a market leading device focused company. To control costs in light of the changing purchasing environment, Medtronic reorganized its cardiovascular division away from a physician-influence focused model to a bids, tender and procurement model. It consolidated its multiple cardiovascular sales and marketing organizations into a centralized cardiovascular business with a single sales force – shifting its focus from physicians to tenders/contract bids and hospital purchasing/administration. The cardiovascular business includes: pacemakers, implantable defibrillators, leads and delivery systems, ablation products, electrophysiology catheters, products for the treatment of atrial fibrillation, information systems for the management of patients with CRDM (Cardiac Rhythm Disease Management) devices, coronary and peripheral stents and related delivery systems, therapies for uncontrolled hypertension, endovascular stent graft systems, heart valve replacement technologies, tissue ablation systems, open heart and coronary bypass grafting surgical products, external defibrillators including manual defibrillator/monitors used by hospitals and emergency response personnel, and automated external defibrillators used in commercial and public settings for the treatment of cardiac arrest. In February 2011, Medtronic terminated five national contracts with Novation for sales of cardiovascular and orthopedic devices – and earlier in the year a national contract for spinal devices with Premier, the second largest GPO (group purchasing organization) behind Novation. Medtronic stated that elimination of the administrative fees paid (generally one- to three-percent) did not appear to help Medtronic grow its market share. Instead, the GPO contract discounted price became the starting price when Medtronic entered into negotiations with hospitals/hospital systems – which it had and has to do with each hospital or hospital system. Medtronic estimated that ending these relationships would save the company $60 million per year.

Medical Device Brand Choice
Shifting From Physicians to Institutions and Patients

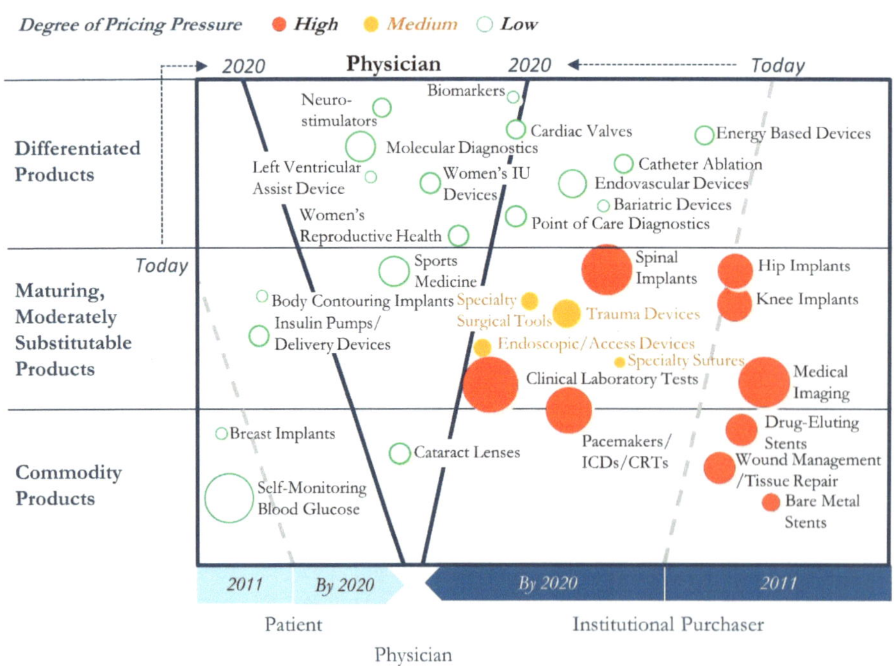

Sources: Adapted by MMC International from U.S. Health Reform: The catalyst to restructure the Life Sciences Industry. By Deloitte.

The migration away from physician specification favors broad product line medical device companies.

When the brand purchase decision shifts from the physician to purchasing/administration or the patient, payers are stating that the product is viewed as equivalent to other marketplace offerings and that decisions will be made largely based upon price. However, in the increasingly sophisticated institutional purchasing environment, price means the total acquisition cost for an item. This means that the true cost of a product is the price paid for the product, the cost related to working with the manufacturer, inventory costs, and the costs associated with getting the product to the patient. It may also include the comparative costs of utilizing the device in patient care. To capture a competitive advantage, large manufacturers bundle their product offerings and may reward the customer for delivering on certain volumes/market shares for certain products. These tactics put limited line manufacturers under pricing pressures to capture business. They are also forced into strategic alliances to tie up complementary products in order to enhance their product offerings/ability to compete. If you are not a market leader, the only effective way to compete is to innovate new differentiable products, which through comparative effectiveness, health care assessment, and outcomes data, show that they improve patient care while decreasing overall treatment costs. Well-served product segments, if not already consolidated, are expected to be consolidated between 2012 and 2020. This trend will favor the largest medical device companies.

Top 100 Medical Device Companies Worldwide In 2010

Johnson & Johnson
General Electric Co.
Siemens AG
Medtronic Inc.
Baxter International Inc.
Koninklijke Philips Electronics NV
Covidien Plc.
Roche Diagnostics
Cardinal Health Inc.
Boston Scientific Corp.
Becton, Dickinson and Co.
Stryker Corp.
Abbott Laboratories
B. Braun Melsungen AG
St. Jude Medical Inc.
Toshiba Corp.
3M Co.
Olympus Corp.
Zimmer Holdings Inc.
Danaher Corp.
Terumo Corp.
Smith & Nephew Plc.
Synthes Inc.
Beckman Coulter Inc.
Alcon Inc.
Getinge AB
Fresenius Medical Care AG & Co. KGaA
C. R. Bard Inc.
Biomet Inc.
Varian Medical Systems Inc.
Carestream Health Inc.
Dentsply International Inc.
Paul Hartmann AG
Alere Inc.
Kinetic Concepts Inc.
Bayer AG
Drägerwerk AG & Co. KGaA
bioMérieux SA
Sonova Holding AG
Invacare Corp.
Hologic Inc.
Coloplast A/S
Nipro Corp.
Agfa-Gevaert NV
Sysmex Corp.
Hill-Rom Holdings Inc.
Kimberly-Clark Corp.
Edwards Lifesciences Corp.
Teleflex Inc.
Intuitive Surgical Inc.
Nihon Kohden Corp.
Hitachi Medical Corp.
Smiths Group Plc.
William Demant Holding A/S
The Cooper Companies Inc.
Fukuda Denshi Co. Ltd.
ResMed Inc.
Konica Minolta Holdings Inc.
Elekta AB
Hospira Inc.
Sorin SpA
Amplifon SpA
Steris Corp.
Carl Zeiss Meditec AG
Allergan Inc.
Sirona Dental Systems Inc.
Nobel Biocare Holding AG
Omron Corp.
Integra LifeSciences Holdings Corp.
Conmed Corp.
Straumann Holding AG
Mindray Medical International Ltd.
Haemonetics Corp.
Cochlear Ltd.
Barco NV
Orthofix International NV
GN Store Nord A/S
Gen-Probe Inc.
American Medical Systems Holdings Inc.
Greatbatch Inc.
Wright Medical Group Inc.
Nikkiso Co. Ltd.
NuVasive Inc.
Zoll Medical Corp.
Analogic Corp.
Masimo Corp.
Align Technology Inc.
Thoratec Corp.
Topcon Corp.
Medical Action Industries Inc.
ArthroCare Corp.
Ansell Ltd.
Symmetry Medical Inc.
Immucor Inc.
Merit Medical Systems Inc.
Volcano Corp.
ICU Medical Inc.
SonoSite Inc.
Cantel Medical Corp.
Horiba Ltd.

There are a myriad of technologies that will transform the medical device industry between 2012 and 2020.

Like the pharmaceutical industry, generic products and substitutable products serve the majority of treatment needs. However, like biotechnology and drugs coupled with biomarkers, there are a myriad of technologies that will enable the medical device industry to upgrade existing medical devices and develop new devices to serve a growing list of unmet medical needs being created by a change to wellness and outcomes-based reimbursement. Nanotechnology, IT/wireless capabilities for hospitals, less invasive surgeries and devices, and combination devices involving drugs and/or biologics are often stated as the hot technology areas for medical devices. However, change is also being fueled by a myriad of other medical device technologies. While the overall medical device industry is in the "maturity" phase of its industry lifecycle, there are significant new opportunities that will revitalize or replace many existing mature products.

Top 20 Medical Device Technologies

1. Stents
2. Capsule Endoscopy
3. Neurostimulation
4. Joint Replacement
5. Neural Interface Systems
6. Ventricular Assist Devices
7. Total Disc Replacement
8. Medical Robotics
9. Percutaneous Aortic Valve
10. Bronchial Thermoplasty
11. Negative Pressure Wound Therapy
12. Natural-orifice transluminal endoscopic surgery
13. Thoracic Endografting
14. Engineered Cartilage Repair Products
15. Musculoskeletal Growth Factors
16. Site Specific Drug Delivery
17. Remote Reporting Implantable Devices
18. Bariatric Surgery
19. Bionic Limbs
20. Cardiac Ablation

Source: Frost and Sullivan presentation.

Medical Device Industry Lifecycle

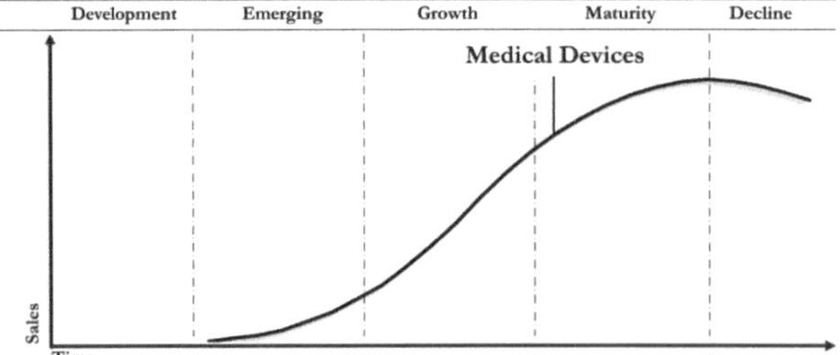

	Development	Emerging	Growth	Maturity	Decline
Risk	Medium	High / Medium	Medium / Low	Low / High	Low
Strategy	Develop Product Portfolio	Secure Market Position	Capture Dominant Market Position	Redeploy Resources (Higher Return Areas)	Focus on Free Cash Flows
Resource Allocation	Invest	Invest	Invest	Maintain/Harvest	Harvest

Source: MMC International.

Companies are restructuring and investing in acquisitions, new product pipelines and/or global expansion.

When an industry is maturing, managements are forced to make tough resource allocation decisions. These generally require new organizational structures to accommodate strategic acquisitions or divestitures. All costs are scrutinized and eliminated where possible. Part of this process is understanding customer success requirements as related to the products sold by the company. The product portfolio and research and development are scrutinized to insure the company will have a sustainable product mix in the future and that the current products are truly profitable. Part of the analysis for global industries is an evaluation of international markets. This is the process strategically-driven device companies have been going through for the last few years. The realization is that significant value can be created by consolidating specific market segments and capturing shared scale economies. It has also become clear that some products which may be considered mature in the developed markets (e.g., United States, European Union countries, and Japan) are finding double digit growth in developing markets, especially in the fast growing BRIC (Brazil, Russia, India, and China) countries with their rapidly expanding middle class with a growing ability to pay for care and the related medical devices. In turn, the companies are extracting costs from their historic organizations through restructurings designed to capitalize on the shifting marketplace. The top twenty medical device companies are especially well positioned to make the changes and investments to prosper from the changing medical device marketplace, not only in the United States but worldwide. Those that maintain or capture a leadership position in their core product areas will create significant corporate and personal wealth and will generate significant free cash flows to fund future growth and expansion.

Top 20 Medical Device Companies
Estimated 2010 Device Sales In Billions of United States Dollars

Rank	Company	2010 Device Sales	Rank	Company	2010 Device Sales
1.	Johnson & Johnson	24.6	16.	3M Healthcare	4.5
2.	GE Healthcare	16.9	17.	Zimmer	4.2
3.	Siemens Healthcare	16.7	18.	Danaher	4.1
4.	Medtronic	15.8	19.	Smith & Nephew	4.0
5.	Baxter International	12.8	20.	Care Fusion	3.9
6.	Philips Healthcare	11.4	21.	Hospira	3.9
7.	Abbott Laboratories	9.3	22.	Olympus Medical	3.9
8.	Cardinal Health	8.8	23.	Synthes	3.7
9.	Covidien	8.4	24.	Beckman Coulter	3.7
10.	Boston Scientific	7.8	25.	Terumo	3.4
11.	Beckton Dickinson	7.4	26.	Alcon	3.2
12.	Stryker	7.3	27.	Fresenius Medical	3.0
13.	B. Braun	5.9	28.	Biomet	2.7
14.	St. Jude Medical	5.2	29.	C.R. Bard	2.7
15.	Toshiba	4.6	30.	Varian Medical	2.4

Source: Medical Products Outsourcing (MCO) magazine. The device and diagnostic companies are ranked according to sales reported for fiscal year 2010 (though some 2011 figures, depending on the fiscal year where possible). Some sales figures may include non-device sales within a division, such as combination products, drug delivery, software or device-related services. Not all companies explicitly break out the device portion of total revenues. MCO consulted numerous public documents and contacted company officials as needed to arrive at the best estimates. Foreign currency conversions were done based on the exchange rate at the end of the fiscal reporting period being discussed.

22 CONCLUSIONS

The Patient Protection and Accountable Care Act (PPACA) is the single largest technology stimulus, innovation implementation and development, job creation, and waste elimination legislation in the history of the United States. It capitalizes on the convergence of a myriad of technologies and utilizes free market competition to begin the elimination of the over $1 trillion in annual United States healthcare system inefficiencies and waste (more than $12.1 trillion between 2012 and 2020). Through legislation, regulation, incentives, pilot programs, grants, penalties, and changes in Medicare reimbursement, it is shifting: 1) provider focus from treatments to preventative care and wellness, and 2) manufacturers' focus from developing products to developing cost-effective medical outcomes.

The fundamental shift in how care is viewed and reimbursed will result in provider consolidations and innovations to extract costs and improve patient care and provider profitability. This will result in healthcare organizations organized around total patient care, prevention, and wellness. The organizations will incorporate physicians and virtually all patient care locations from home care to hospital care. This will lead to fewer but larger purchasers. As the power shifts from physicians to payers, purchasing and healthcare administrators, how products are specified and purchased will be transformed. These changes are resulting in focus shifts and power shifts throughout the $2.6 trillion (2010) United States healthcare industry. As a result, virtually all participants are innovating to protect or grow their revenues, market shares and profitability. This has thrust all industry stakeholders into a period of discontinuity where traditional ways of doing business are being, will be replaced by new, emerging industry norms – often changing industry boundaries.

The shift from purchasing products to value purchasing will revitalize many healthcare industry product markets. The focus of research and development investments will be on developing truly unique product offerings that objectively and cost-effectively deliver better patient outcomes along with attractive margins. This will result in a shift from investing in me-too products to investments in unique products, many of which will have global markets. Since most products are equivalent or substitutable products (commodity products), price competition will intensify in the United States. This has and will continue to prompt industry segment consolidations as well as an increased focus on international markets, especially the BRIC (Brazil, Russia, India, and China) markets. The fast-growing middle classes in the BRIC countries increasingly have the ability to pay for the commodity products as well as new innovative products. Internationalization increases revenues from the current product portfolios and establishes the marketing infrastructure for the innovative products that will be developed in the future – creating United States jobs.

Periods of industry discontinuity are the best times to create corporate and personal wealth. The degree of discontinuity will be healthcare industry segment and company dependent. Generic strategies will not work. Managements have to create and execute their unique strategies using objective critical analysis based upon facts. Strategically-managed companies will be handsomely rewarded. Those that fail to adapt and/or execute will be broken up, acquired, merged or driven out of business.

The multi-trillion dollars available for cost sharing through the elimination of United States healthcare industry waste is unprecedented. It will lead to a U.S. healthcare gold rush between 2012 and 2020 which will create significant corporate and personal wealth.

ABOUT THE AUTHOR

Edmund L. Valentine has over 27 years of global healthcare industry experience. He has been the editor of multiple editions of MMC International's *Trends Shaping U.S. Pharmaceutical Industry Strategies* reports as well as therapeutic area reviews. Valentine is Chairman and C.E.O. of MMC International, a strategy, general management, business development, marketing and technology assessment advisory firm primarily focusing on the global healthcare industry. He is a recognized authority on the trends shaping the U.S. healthcare system.

www.ingramcontent.com/pod-product-compliance
Lightning Source LLC
LaVergne TN
LVHW070953210926
848482LV00002B/198

9780984047802